W9-CDF-751

An Atlas of Overdentures and Attachments

by

Joseph F. Jumber, D.D.S.

In collaboration with
Michael J. Jumber, D.M.D.
and Frank H. Anderson, D.D.S.

quintessence
books

Quintessence Publishing Co., Inc.   1981
Chicago, Berlin, Rio de Janeiro, Tokyo

© 1981 by Quintessence Publishing Co., Inc., Chicago, Illinois.
All rights reserved.

This book or any part thereof must not be reproduced by any means or in any
form without the written permission of the publisher.

Lithography: Industrie- und Presseklischee, Berlin.
Composition: Adolph Fürst & Sohn GmbH & Co., Typographische Anstalt, Berlin.
Printing: Universal Printing Company, St. Louis.
Binding: Becktold Company, St. Louis.
Printed in the U.S.A.

ISBN 0-931386-06-3

This book is dedicated to my loving
wife Irene . . .
He made only one like her
and I was lucky to have found her.
Thanks for 30 wonderful years.
And in memory of
Sara Michelle Jumber
(October 2-9, 1979)

Foreword

It is an honor and a welcomed privilege to be asked to write the foreword for this excellent book. I know of no one who is more competent than Joe Jumber to explain the intricacies and the wide range of options associated with overdenture prostheses. His experience in both the clinical and the technical aspects of restorative treatment makes Dr. Jumber uniquely qualified to explain the rationale as well as the techniques of overdenture fabrication.

The conscientious dentist of today is dedicated to the preservation of every tooth that can be maintained in health. Even loose teeth with considerable loss of bone support can serve a useful role in stabilizing and retaining a removable prosthesis. The added security and comfort to the patient certainly warrants special attention to save and use teeth that a few years ago would have been considered hopeless. In attempting to use periodontally weak teeth as abutments for prosthetic replacement of missing teeth, the dentist must rely on sound basic principles but must also have a wide variety of treatment options. The overdenture is one option that should be selected with care and understanding.

There are as many ways to use overdentures as there are patients, so it is important to understand that when overdenture treatment is the method selected, it does not simply involve making a full denture to fit over roots. The success or failure of many overdentures depends on subtle differences in design or fabrication. It is far more involved with crown and bridge procedures than with conventional full denture prosthetics. Predictable success in overdenture prosthetics requires an involvement in periodontics, endodontics and precision attachment prosthetics, as well as basic restorative procedures.

With most overlay procedures, the use of precision attachments can be beneficial. Proper selection of the right attachment is often the difference between a simple, reliable prosthesis compared with one that is far too complicated. Failure to select the right attachment for each situation almost always adds to the complexity. The step-by-step explanation of many different procedures makes this atlas a very valuable reference work as it describes the techniques for using many different types of attachment-retained prostheses as well as simple coping or bar retention.

The descriptions and explanations of every aspect of overdenture construction should be invaluable for both the dentist and the technician. This atlas should enable the careful dentist to serve many patients with an alternative that is far superior to conventional complete dentures.

Peter E. Dawson, D.D.S.

7

Preface

A person is fortunate indeed when he has all of his teeth and enjoys the benefits of a healthy, normal oral cavity. For many persons, the onslaught of caries and periodontal disease soon destroys their teeth, and periodontium. Unfortunately, many such patients, rather than save their teeth, have them removed and replaced with complete dentures. Yes! Too often the patient is not informed that such teeth can still be retained for many years. Often it is a simple matter to keep his teeth for many years with sound restorative procedures and periodontal therapy.

As teeth are lost, the remaining teeth may shift from their original positions, and teeth opposite the edentulous areas extrude downward or supraerupt. There is a general collapse of the dental arches, as well as periodontal problems associated with such changes in the dentition. As these problems continue, the patient may even experience typical temporomandibular joint problems. Of course, if adequate teeth and bone support remain, many of these problems can be eliminated by restoring the dentition with a fixed or removable prosthesis. However, as time passes, the dentition may be subjected to extreme bone loss associated with very advanced periodontal disease. When many teeth are missing, a situation which appears to be generally hopeless may exist. Only minimal bone may be supporting the remaining teeth. Now, to utilize these remaining teeth safely as abutments to support some form of fixed bridgework –

such as a periodontal splint, or even a combination of fixed bridgework and precision partial dentures – would be hazardous. Complete dentures should always be the last resort.

When utilizing teeth with a questionable prognosis, the eventual loss of a key tooth may jeopardize the function and usefulness of the entire dental treatment. Therefore, in extreme situations in which there is extensive bone loss around the remaining teeth, or in which there are only a few teeth, routine types of restorative dentistry may be contraindicated. An overlay prosthesis such as an overdenture may now be the treatment of choice.

An overdenture may be defined as a prosthetic replacement of the natural dentition that covers retained vital or non-vital teeth or the roots of teeth. The utilization of teeth to support an overlay prosthesis is not a new technique. It is a procedure that has been used by earlier practitioners for many years. Recently, overdenture prosthodontics has experienced a renewed popularity. Unfortunately many dentists are misled by the term "overdenture" and feel that this treatment is similar to complete denture treatment. I often hear the comment: "I don't make dentures." As a result, patients whose teeth can still be saved are referred elsewhere for complete denture treatment. Such patients are unnecessarily forced into the remainder of their lifetime with the problems associated with complete dentures. This is unfortunate since overdenture prosthodontics, as practiced by the authors, is actually crown and bridge prosthodontics including a tremendous amount of all phases of dental treatment such as periodontics, endodontics, crown restorations and attachment-retained prosthesis.

In speaking to and working with many dentists and laboratory technicians in seminars and participatory clinics on overdentures, it soon became apparent that there was a need for a complete and thorough step-by-step guide covering in detail all clinical and laboratory procedures that would facilitate the effective management of even the most extreme dental situations.

However, the authors feel that overdenture prosthodontics is not necessarily a technique requiring treatment by only a specialist with "special training." These techniques are readily managed by the serious student of restorative dentistry.

With that in mind, this book was organized to guide the dentist and technician through the various phases of overdenture prosthodontics.

It was also apparent that treatment planning seemed to be a difficult area of overdenture prosthodontics. Included is a complete chapter on treatment planning that should help the practitioner to develop a suitable treatment for his patients. It should also help in the coordination of the clinical and laboratory phases of such treatment.

Although the purpose of this text is not to teach endodontics or periodontics, these dental procedures are an indispensable part of overdenture treatment. There is outlined a simple approach to conventional endodontics. Most patients considered for such overdenture treatment have advanced periodontal disease. Restoration of the oral apparatus should never be attempted without considering the health of the periodontium. As the success or failure of restorative treatment may be directly related to the health of the periodontium, the authors tried to emphasize the extreme importance between the relationship of

coping design and embrasure form as they relate to periodontal health. We consider this as one of the more important sections of this book.

Most teeth used as overdenture abutments have minimal bone support. These teeth must be reduced to form a favorable crown to root ratio which decreases destructive lateral forces. Since copings fitted on such short abutments have minimal retention, we have presented numerous techniques for providing auxiliary retention to retain the copings on their abutments.

Overdentures may be supported on bare roots with or without attachments, or on coping-restored roots designed for just support or fitted with attachments for retention. The authors feel that overlay prostheses should have many of the important features of crown and bridge – precision partial prosthetics. Therefore the authors have included numerous chapters covering a wide range of overdenture types and attachments. The use of overdenture attachments and step-by-step procedures in their fabrication make up a large portion of this text. We have tried to simplify attachment selection by stressing the importance of understanding basic principles applicable to attachment use.

It is not convenient within the limits of this text to discuss and illustrate all attachments available for use in overdenture prosthodontics. However, we have tried especially hard to cover in complete detail all clinical and laboratory steps in the use and fabrication of many of the commonly used overdenture attachments. The chapters on specific attachments should be of tremendous aid to the laboratory technicians who must fabricate the prosthesis, as well as the dentist who should thoroughly understand the attachments' function and their fabrication. Without this knowledge, the dentist's success in overdenture treatment and maintenance will be compromised.

It is the authors' personal wish that this text

will help dentists perceive alternate treatments for patients other than the complete denture.

Any work such as this is not the result of a few individuals efforts but it is due to the unselfish contribution from many during one's professional lifetime. Such influence is often difficult to identify and to isolate. The seed is often planted and nourished from a patient's dental and emotional needs; from attendance at many seminars; by reading texts authored by dedicated clinicians who have laid the groundwork through their vision and energetic and unselfish contributions to dental education, and yes, from personal contact with many colleagues who in some manner have touched and left me with their lasting influence.

This personal relationship was started early in my dental education. As a student, I was deeply indebted to Dr. Arthur George, Dr. Merle Christy and Mr. Joe Sakmar. Their enthusiasm in teaching and desire for perfection helped to arouse my interest in prosthodontics.

Early in my dental practice I was fortunate to meet Dr. Frank Scott. His unselfish dedication to his patients, fellow dentists and personal commitment to ideal dentistry have been a great source of personal motivation. His never-ceasing encouragement has been a constant source of professional energy.

It is indeed unusual when a dentist is not touched and influenced in some manner by Dr. L. D. Pankey. Such an individual, with his understanding of human nature and life in general, must certainly occur rarely in a lifetime. His excellent seminars have been a tremendous influence on my attitude toward my family and my patients.

Dr. Henry Ebel has been a source of tremendous help and encouragement. He is one who gave unselfishly of his time and specialized knowledge. His understanding of the principles of prosthodontics was always a source of help and guidance. He was a very gracious and helpful influence in formulating my thinking throughout the development of this text.

Dr. Peter Dawson is one of those individuals with the unique ability to clearly analyze a patient's problem and develop a practical approach to treating these patients for ideal comfort, function and esthetics. His ability to transfer this knowledge to others has been a tremendous aid to me personally, and to dentistry in general.

The peridontal health of many of the patients described in this text is due to the excellent periodontal surgery and management performed by Dr. Frank Scott, Dr. Walter Watson, Dr. Richard Miller, Dr. Harold Pattishall, Dr. Robert Romans, Dr. Jack Whitman and Dr. Lamar Pearson. I am grateful for their cooperation and pleasant association.

Dr. Henry Holton, Dr. Jerry Stoddard, Dr. Fred Mann and Dr. Jerry Rothstein have been especially helpful in the treatment of special surgical problems associated with many of my patients.

Having the opportunity of treating numerous cleft palate patients in cooperation with Dr. Neal Roth and Dr. Richard Skinner has been a rewarding experience. Their unselfish help and guidance have given me a deeper appreciation of the value of overdenture prosthodontics. I am grateful for it.

A special and warm feeling of appreciation is felt for Dr. Warren Rhunau and Mrs. Glenda Rhunau, Dr. Gordon Perkins and Dr. Donald Sitterson for the opportunity of treating many of their patients.

I have learned much about overdenture treatment from discussions with Dr. Bernard Swafford, Dr. Philip Abood and Dr. Merrill Mensor. It is appreciated.

The development of this manuscript in its present form would have been impossible without the unselfish and dedicated efforts of Mr. David Selander. His grasp of an unfamiliar subject and ability to reorganize some of my efforts into a more readable form has always been an amazement to me. Dave, I'll be forever grateful.

Thanks!

Mr. Carlos James has taught me much of what I know of photography.

Mr. Thomas Bormes, Mr. Carl Miller and Mr. Phillip Larson have also added to the improvement of this text. Their knowledge of attachments has been extremely helpful.

I am especially indebted to my friend and neighbor Marion Probst. I owe so much for her unselfish help and enthusiasm in typing the manuscript many, many times. Completing the manuscript would have been difficult without her help. Thank you, Marion!

A special thanks to Mr. Harold Sigmon who has helped in many ways.

I am also grateful to Dr. Alvin Fillastre, Dr. Henry Collette, Dr. Carl Hermann Voss, Dr. John Tallent and Mr. Jim Ward for their help in editing this manuscript.

It would be impossible to treat a patient satisfactorily without the aid of a competent staff. Technicians Mrs. Delphine McGee, Mr. Mike Foster, Mr. Joel Murphy and Mr. Chet Simmons have made my task easier and more enjoyable.

Special acknowledgement is due Dr. Richard Chaikin for his kind advice and for accepting this book for publication; to Mr. H. W. Haase, the publisher, who made this book a reality; and to Mr. Peter Sielaff with whom it was so enjoyable to work with in the production of this book. This book is the result of the efforts and influence of many others. I feel very grateful to those not mentioned, especially the many dentists of Northeastern Florida who have made this area a most enjoyable one in which to practice.

Joseph F. Jumber

Contents

Foreword 7

Preface 9

Chapter 1
**Why Select Overdentures Instead
of Complete Dentures** 17

Debilitated Oral Conditions 17
Alveolar Bone Loss and the
Complete Denture 17
The Value of Retaining Roots 17
A Different Philosophy for
'Hopeless Teeth' 17
The Overlay Prosthesis 20
Advantages of Overdentures 20
  Superior Method of Treatment 20
  Conservation of the
  Alveolar Ridge 20
  Conservation of the Remaining
  Abutments 20
  Prosthesis Stability 20
  Retention 21
  Esthetics 21
  More Stable Occlusion 21
  Open Palates 22
  Proprioceptive Response 22
  Distribution of Forces of Mastication 22
  Fewer Denture Adjustments 22
  Easily Modified to Complete
  Dentures 22
Disadvantages of Overdentures 22
  Cost 22
  Overdenture Bulk 23
  Overdenture and Patient
  Considerations 23

Chapter 2
Examination and Diagnosis 25

Examination 25
  Patient History 25

Study Casts – An Aid to
Treatment Planning 25
Clinical Examination 25
Radiographic Examination 26
Diagnosis 26
  Evaluation and Selection of
  Abutments (for Overdentures) 26
  Abutment Location 26
  Bone Support 27
  Proximal Space Between
  Abutments 27
  Number of Teeth Available 29
  Masticatory Load and the
  Opposing Dentition 29
  Design of the Prosthesis 29

Chapter 3
Treatment Planning 31

Treatment of Multiple Problems 31
Coordination of Multiple Treatments 31
  Will Special Surgical
  Procedures or Extractions
  be Necessary? 31
  Will Periodontal Surgery
  be Necessary? 31
  Will Endodontics
  be Necessary? 31
  Will an Interim Overdenture be
  Necessary? 32
Various Categories of Patients with
Multiple Dental Problems 32
  Overdenture Condition I 32
  Overdenture Condition II 32
  Overdenture Condition III 33
Treatment Plan Sequence 34
  Examination 35
  Prophylaxis 35
Operative Appointment No. 1 36
  Root Reduction 36
  Endodontic Therapy 36
  Extractions 39

Contents

Periodontal Surgery	39
Operative Appointment No. 2	41
Operative Appointment No. 3	41
Abutment Preparations	41
Impressions	42
Operative Appointment No. 4	42
Try-in of the Castings	42
Master Overdenture Impressions	42
Operative Appointment No. 5	42
Occlusal Registration	42
Operative Appointment No. 6	42
Operative Appointment No. 7	43
Cementation	43
Home Care Instructions	43

Chapter 4
Abutment and Coping Considerations — **45**

General Abutment Consideration	45
Coping Types	45
Long Copings	45
Medium Copings	48
Medium-Short Copings	48
Short Copings	48
The Relation of Coping Type to Alveolar Support and Vitality	50

Chapter 5
Endodontics — **51**

Endodontics Before Operative Appointment	51
Endodontics during Initial Operative Appointment	51
Providing Access	51
Treating Many Roots at One Time	52
Instrumentation and Length Control	53
Pin-Grid Length Control Instrumentation Techniques	53
Procedure for Rapid Endodontics	53
Mechanical Instrumentation	54
Root Canal Irrigation and Medication	56
Root Canal Obturation	56

Chapter 6
Periodontics and the Overdenture — **61**

Periodontal Consideration	61
Periodontal Therapy Prior to the Operative Appointments	62
Periodontal Therapy during Operative Appointments	64
Periodontal Surgery sometime after Extractions	64
Treatment of the most Common Periodontal Condition	64
Periodontal Therapy	65
Periodontal Surgery Management with Interim Overdentures	67
Interim Overdentures, Vital Abutments and Periodontal Management	68

Chapter 7
Interim or Transitional Overdentures — **69**

Management Techniques	69
Functions of Interim Overdentures	69
Modification of Existing Prosthesis	69
Immediate Interim Overdenture Using Denture Teeth	73
Other Interim Overdenture Considerations	74

Chapter 8
Abutment Preparations and Coping Consideration — **75**

Short Preparation for Bare-Root Abutment	76
Short Preparation for Short Copings	76
Medium-Short Preparation with Non-Vital Teeth	77
Medium-Short Preparations for Bare-Root Abutments	78
Medium-Short Preparations for Copings	78
Medium Coping Preparation for Vital or Non-Vital Teeth	81
Long Preparations with Vital Teeth	81
Long Primary Coping Preparations for Use with an Acrylic Resin Secondary Coping	81
Preparations for Long Primary Coping to be Used with Metal Secondary Copings	83

Chapter 9
Coping Retention — **85**

Dowel (Post) Retention	85
Non-Parallel Posts	85
Parallel Post	85
The Para-Post System for Parallel Canal Preparations	86
Basic Materials for Para-Post Dowels and Pin Retention	86
Pin Materials	87
Para-Post Procedure for Parallel Post Canals	89
Other Post Systems	89
Stutz Pivot	92
Schenker Stepped Pivot	92

Parallel Pins   93
    Condition of Teeth   93
    Parallel Pin Technique   93
Post-Pin Retention   94
    With Splinted Copings   94
    With Separate Single Copings   94

Chapter 10
Impressions – Casts –
Occlusal Registration   99

Impressions   99
Custom Trays   99
Abutment Impressions and Casts   102
Overdenture Impressions and Casts   105
    Substructure Cemented on
    Abutments   105
    Casts with Substructure "Pulled" with
    Impression   105
    Casts with Substructure Cemented
    Using Transfer Males   105
Cast Orientation   106
    Articulation of Casts for Coping
    Fabrication and Attachments   106
    Orientation of Casts for Overdenture
    Fabrication   106
Record Bases   106
    Stabilized Wax or Shellac Record
    Bases   106
    Resin Bases   106
    Framework Record Bases   107
Occlusal Registration   107
    Functionally Generated Occlusal
    Technique   107

Chapter 11
Waxed Patterns and Coping
Consideration   113

Coping Consideration   113
    Coping Patterns for Periodontal
    Health   113
    Coping Patterns for Esthetics   116
    Coping Patterns for Stability and
    Support   116
    Coping Patterns for Retention   116
    Coping Patterns for Stud Attachments 116
    Coping Patterns for Bar Attachments 119
    Coping Patterns for Auxiliary
    Attachments   119
    Waxing Procedure   119

Chapter 12
Overdenture Framework   123

Maxillary Design   123

Major Connector   123
Minor Connector   126
Mandibular Design   126
    Major Connector   126
General Considerations   126

Chapter 13
Overdenture Design   133

Bare Root Overdenture   133
Telescopic Overdenture   133
Attachment Fixation Overdenture   135
Superiority of Attachment-Fixation
Overdenture   135
    Attachment Selection   135
    Resilient or Non-Resilient
    Attachments   136
    Extra-Coronal Attachment Selection   138
    Bar Attachments Selection   138
    Stud Attachment Selection   142
    Auxiliary Attachment Selection   142

Chapter 14
Telescopic Overdenture   145

Advantages and Disadvantages of
Telescopic Overdentures   145
    Advantages   145
    Disadvantages   145
    Overdenture Function   146
Coping Design   146
A Telescopic Overdenture Treatment   146
    Procedure   146
Relining and/or Rebasing   152

Chapter 15
The Zest Anchor Attachment   153

The Attachment   153
    Attachment Function   153
    Zest Anchor Components   153
    Zest Overdenture Procedure   155
Basic Technique   155
    Indirect Procedure   155
    Root Preparation and Seating of
    Females   156
    Indirect Procedure for Processing
    Males into the Denture   158
    Direct Technique   163
    Indirect Procedure Using Gold
    Copings   165
    Gold Coping Procedure   165
Mini-Zest Anchorage   167
    Procedures   167

Contents

Relining and Rebasing Procedures	169
Rebasing Procedures	169
Replacement of Broken Male Posts	171
Miscellaneous Uses for the Zest	171
Trouble-shooting with Zest Anchor	171

Chapter 16
Bar Attachments **173**

Types for Bar Attachments	173
The Bar Unit	173
The Bar Joint	173
The Dolder Bar	175
Typical Dolder Bar Treatment	175
Overdenture Function	183
Adjusting Retention	183
Relining/Rebasing Technique	183
The Dolder Bar Unit	185
General Technique	185
Other Bar Systems	185
Customized Bars	186
Retentive Clips Used with	
Customized Bars	188
The Hader Bar System	191
Components of Attachment	191
Hader Bar Technique	191
Relining/Rebasing the Hader Bar	
System	193

Chapter 17
Stud Attachments **195**

Stud Anchorage Systems	195
When to Use a Stud Attachment	195
When to Use a Resilient Stud	195
When to Use a Non-Resilient Stud	
Attachment	197
Some Stud Attachments	197
The Gerber Attachment and its Functions	199
Resilient Gerber Overdenture	
Treatment	199
Examination, Diagnosis and	
Treatment Planning	199
Clinical and Technical Procedures	199
Step-by-Step Technique	200

Non-Resilient Gerber	207
Maintenance Consideration	207
Some Characteristics of the Gerber	
Attachment	211
Dalla Bona Attachment	211
Cylindrical Dalla Bona	211
Spherical Dalla Bona	213
Advantages	213
Disadvantages	213
Spherical Dalla Bona Treatment	213
Processing the Female Attachment	
at Chairside	215
The Rotherman Attachment	219
Rotherman Overdenture Treatment	219
Some Advantages of the Rotherman	220
Some Disadvantages of	
the Rotherman	223
Relining or Rebasing of the	
Rotherman	223
Miscellaneous Stud Attachments	227
Ancrofix Attachment	227
Introfix and Gmur Attachments	227
Bona-Puffer Stud	228

Chapter 18
Auxiliary Attachments **229**

Screws	229
Screw Attachments	229
Schubiger Screw Attachment	229
The Schubiger Technique	229
Plunger-Type Attachments	231
Ipsoclip and Presso-matic	
Attachments	231
IC Attachment	234

Chapter 19
Overdenture Maintenance
and Oral Health **239**

Overdenture Instructions	239
Substructure and Abutment Instructions	241
Bibliography	245
Subject Index	249

Chapter 1

Why Select Overdentures Instead of Complete Dentures

In most instances overdentures are a superior alternative to a routine type of complete denture supported only by the alveolar tissues.

Debilitated Oral Conditions

During the patient's examination, you may find that the dentition has advanced periodontal disease. There may be numerous teeth missing, extreme caries may be present and often the teeth literally are covered with thick layers of calculus. Never make your diagnosis based on the hopeless appearance presented by such a broken-down dentition (Figs. 1a to d). A few teeth may have fair supporting bone structure while others have no bone support at all, being held in place with just epithelium. In such a situation, examine every tooth thoroughly to determine if the tooth or root can be successfully used to support and retain an overdenture.

Alveolar Bone Loss and the Complete Denture

The main function of alveolar bone is to house the roots of teeth. Rapid bone resorption may occur if teeth are removed. The degree of the residual ridge resorption is determined by many local and systemic factors. Generally, the greater the degree of abuse to the alveolar ridge, the more rapid and more extensive the resorption. Since tooth or root retention equals alveolar bone preservation, there is a need for patient education – the decision is theirs.

The Value of Retaining Roots

If the last few remaining teeth or their roots can be saved and used as abutments to support an overdenture, the future loss of the alveolar ridge can be minimized. These teeth will stabilize the overdentures and may even be used to add retention (Figs. 2a to d). Roots retained in the alveolar ridge also tend to conserve the supporting bone adjacent to the neighboring teeth (Fig. 1-3).

A Different Philosophy for 'Hopeless Teeth'

The principles and concepts of overdentures should be added to the armamentarium of the Dentist. The usefulness of such teeth often is based on the dentist's previous education, post-graduate training, experience and judgment – and even, his mental attitude. On the past, when the dentition looked hopeless, extractions and complete dentures were generally considered. Now, however, a complete new philosophy of treatment planning should be considered by the dentist. Such teeth may be hopeless for routine restorative procedures, but they may serve as excellent abutments for overlay prosthodontic appliances.

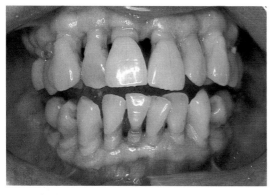

Figs. 1-1a to d   So-called "hopeless" dentitions when overdentures are the treatment of choice. The teeth have multiple dental problems; often many teeth are missing; there is advanced periodontal disease associated with extensive alveolar destruction, and some teeth may have little or no bone support and must be removed. When such oral conditions exist, a diagnosis and treatment plan must not be based solely on the poor general appearance.

Figure 1-1a

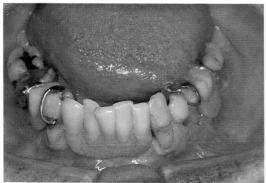

Figure 1-1b

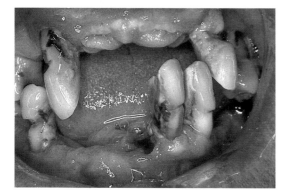

Figure 1-1c

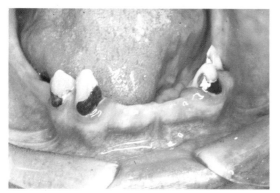

Figure 1-1d

Figs. 1-2a to d "Hopeless" dentitions used as abutments to support overdentures. These abutments may be used without attachments, with attachments placed in bare roots, restored with plain copings, or used with copings and attachments to support and retain an overlay prosthesis.

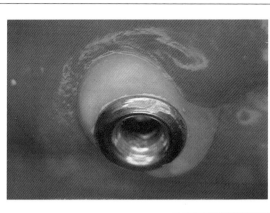

Figure 1-2a

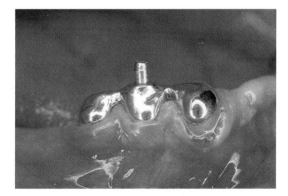

Figure 1-2b

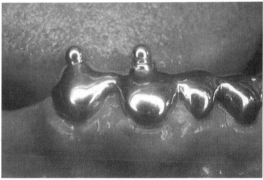

Figure 1-2c

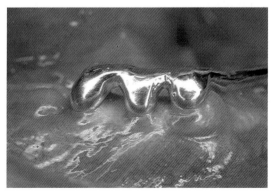

Figure 1-2d

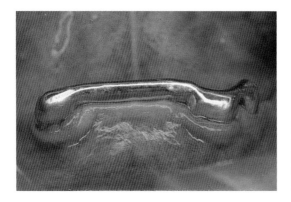

Fig. 1-3 Retained roots conserve the alveolar ridge between abutments as well as some distance distal. Loss of these few remaining teeth would soon result in rapid resorption of the remaining alveolar ridge.

The Overlay Prosthesis

One should never underestimate the usefulness of these so-called "questionable teeth" or their roots to support some form of removable prosthesis.

Teeth or roots of teeth that may be "hopeless" or at least "questionable" for routine restorative procedures, may have an excellent prognosis when used for overlay prosthesis. One can change the prognosis of teeth by varying the treatment plan.

Advantages of Overdentures

Superior Method of Treatment

When the patient has only a few teeth with minimal bone support, conventional fixed bridgework puts all of the forces of mastication on these few weak abutments. An overlay prosthesis has a broader distribution of functional and parafunctional forces, distributing these forces more uniformly over the remaining abutments and surrounding soft tissues. In special conditions such as a cleft-palate – where there may be misalignment of the alveolar ridges, malposed or depressed teeth, or other anatomical defects – an overdenture may be the ideal treatment.

Conservation of the Alveolar Ridge

As mentioned earlier, root retention equals alveolar bone conservation and it is the most important reason for retaining teeth to support an overlay prosthesis.

Conservation of the Remaining Abutments

Weak, loose and mobile teeth – caused by inadequate bone support, poor tooth contact, unfavorable crown-root ratio and misdirected forces of mastication – contribute to bone loss and tooth mobility. Overlay prosthetic treatment brings many of these damaging conditions under control. Reducing these teeth to form a more favorable crown-root ratio, the supporting and splinting effect of the overlay prosthesis and the development of a favorable occlusion distributed over a wider area, help to strengthen and support teeth for many more years of function.

Prosthesis Stability

Conventional complete dentures are retained in part by their broad tissue coverage, flange extension and tissue undercuts. A removable overlay prosthesis, on the other hand, can be retained by the remaining root or tooth abutments. Many of the retained roots are simply reduced to the

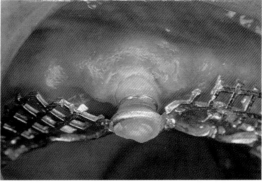

Fig. 1-4 Overdenture framework fitted with attachments and snapped on the abutments. Such root-supported and retained frameworks (used as the occlusal registration trays) provide more accurate occlusal records.

level of the alveolar ridge and utilized strictly for stability of the appliance, with or without copings. Bare roots can be fitted with special retentive attachments or these roots can be restored with long, medium or short copings.

Retention

The copings can also be provided with various types of retentive devices to give added retention to the removable prosthesis.

Whenever possible, this important feature of retention should be considered to increase patient comfort and function. True, retention may not be as important as some of the other benefits of an overlay prosthesis (e.g., stability and preservation of the alveolar ridge); however, it can play a significant part in the patient's acceptance of the prosthesis. A patient should expect this important feature of the removable prosthesis, unless to do so would jeopardize abutments or treatment.

Esthetics

There is more latitude in the design concept of overdentures for maximum improvement in esthetics. When the supporting abutments provide retention for the overlay appliance, flange extensions, so necessary

in complete dentures, are not as mandatory with the overlay prosthesis.

When there are anatomical deformities, such as a cleft-palate or tori, the design of an overlay prosthesis can be much truer to the esthetic qualities of the natural dentition.

More Stable Occlusion

There are not the occlusal recording problems as when working with edentulous resilient tissues. When a removable prosthesis is stabilized and retained by an abutment-supported substructure, a more stable occlusion is possible. By utilizing a root-supported occlusal registration tray, the dentist can obtain more accurate occlusal records. The metal framework used for the final overlay prosthesis can often be fitted with the companion connector attachment and then snapped on to the temporarily or permanently cemented coping substructure. This produces a firm, tooth-connected and stabilized occlusal registation tray (Fig. 1-4).

As such a framework can be secured firmly with the attachments and supported by the abutment teeth, there is no limit to the type of occlusal records obtainable. For example, in addition to the centric occlusal records, one can easily develop ideal customized incisal guidance, plane of occlusion, programmed cuspal inclinations and functionally generated path records, as well as gnathological recordings.

Open Palates

When the overlay prosthesis is retained by an adequate number of maxillary teeth, the appliance needs only minimal palatal coverage. Such open palate overdentures are more successful when the abutments are evenly distributed anteriorly and posteriorly. Thus, when an anatomical deformity is present – such as tori or bony undercuts – the overlay prosthesis can be designed to circumvent these anatomical structures.

Proprioceptive Response

There is a more efficient neuromuscular coordination. An overlay prosthesis supported by abutment teeth feels more natural to the patient than a conventional complete denture due to the increased proprioceptive responses. As he chews, the patient senses the stimulation of the peridontal ligaments attached to the roots. Thus, there is more patient acceptance and greater confidence in his ability to eat, drink and speak.

Distribution of Forces of Mastication

Overdentures distribute forces of mastication more uniformly over the roots and denture-supporting soft tissues. This causes less trauma to the supporting tissues, reducing the alveolar bone resorption normally experienced with complete dentures. By decreasing the crown-root ratio of a tooth, forces of mastication can be directed more directly along the long axis of the tooth, thus reducing damaging lateral forces.

Fewer Denture Adjustments

Another advantage of overdentures is the noticeable decrease in the number of den-

ture adjustments. In fact, the overdenture is normally accepted very well by the patient, with minimal problems. Often it is difficult to persuade the patient to return for his regular recall visits.

Easily Modified to Complete Dentures

Another important advantage of the overlay prosthesis is the ease of modification, should any of the abutment teeth fail. It is an excellent transitional or provisional denture. In fact, it is this important feature which helps to motivate patients to accept overdenture treatment, rather than complete dentures. Even if all abutment teeth are later lost, the overlay prosthesis can generally be modified to act as a complete denture.

Disadvantages of Overdentures

When considering the disadvantages of an overdenture, one must remember with what the comparisons are being made: Overdentures should be reserved for those conditions in which routine crown and bridge procedures are contraindicated. The only other alternative treatment would be complete dentures. In this sense there are no disadvantages to overdentures. All of the problems associated with the overlay technique are minor compared to those problems faced by the totally edentulous patient. However, there are a few aspects of overdentures that could be considered as disadvantages.

Cost

Because overdentures cost more than traditional dentures, added expense involved is a definite disadvantage. Often a more favorable crown-root ratio is desirable. Now reduction of the tooth is mandatory; thus endodontics may or may not be necessary. The abutments can be retained with or without crowns. When copings – with or without attachments – are placed on these roots, the fee, of course, would increase accordingly.

Overdenture Bulk

Occasionally, an overdenture may be bulkier than a complete denture, particularly with a telescopic overlay prosthesis. This can be minimized by reducing the clinical crowns (produces a more favorable crown-root ratio) to provide more room to accommodate the overlay prosthesis. Selection of a specific attachment for the space available helps to control the appliance bulk.

Overdenture and Patient Considerations

There may be more maintenance problems with overdentures:

a) Copings become loose.
b) Attachment wear, loss and breakage.
c) Alveolar ridge resorption.
d) Overdenture breakage.
e) Patient maintenance problems.
f) Patient oral hygiene problems.

Many of these problems can be minimized by proper patient motivation and instruction, treatment planning, and attachment selection.

Chapter 2

Examination and Diagnosis

Examination

Probably the most difficult initial problem faced by the dentist is making an accurate diagnosis to determine if overdenture techniques are indicated or whether the problems can be best solved with alternate restorative procedures. This may be a grey area of diagnosis and treatment planning for there can be more than one treatment plan that can solve a particular problem. But we must consider the treatment that is best for each particular patient, dependent upon our findings.

Patient History

No examination is complete without the complete history of the patient's medical background, psychological evaluation and past dental history. The medical history should be thorough and, when deemed necessary, the patient's physician should be consulted concerning the general health of the patient. The patient should be questioned concerning his past dental treatment and experiences. This dental history should reveal information about the patient's past experience with previous removable appliances, patient's attitude toward his teeth, as well as his home care habits.

Study Casts – An Aid to Treatment Planning

Study casts, properly mounted with accurate occlusal records on an appropriate articulator, provide much needed data: the occlusal relationship of the teeth and arches; the vertical spaces between the arches; the presence or absence of any anatomical structures; and the location of bony undercuts (Fig. 2-1). The study casts will also help determine the amount of tooth reduction necessary, the type of copings to be selected; and, in most cases, the best attachment that can be used for each specific condition. Accurate study casts can also be used for the fabrication of interim overdentures when these are necessary. Duplicate casts can be used for construction of custom trays, Omnavac shells, legal patient record of prior treatment, etc.

Clinical Examination

A clinical examination should start with a complete examination of the entire oral cavity. Carefully examine all of the soft tissue areas for any pathological problems or soft tissue variations. Thoroughly examine the face and neck areas and lymph nodes.

The edentulous ridge areas should be palpated to determine the presence of any loose or flabby tissue and sharp bony ridges; bony protruberances, such as torri, exostosis, or hyperplastic tissues, which might interfere with long-term partial or denture uses. Such areas should be corrected surgically acceptance of the removable prosthesis.

All remaining teeth should be thoroughly examined. This will help to determine the patient's oral hygiene habits, which, if inadequate, should be modified through education before the start of dental treatment. The presence of extensive caries may indicate dietary, caries rate and oral hygiene problems, which will cause failure of the overdenture treatment through recurrent decay.

The occlusal relationship of the teeth, arch form and arch relationship should be studied and evaluated in conjunction with the mounted study casts. Any habits, such as tongue thrust, bruxism, teeth clenching, tongue or lip-biting, should be observed and evaluated to indicate their effect on the long-range success of the dental treatment.

Most patients who are candidates for overdenture treatment have periodontal disease; therefore a thorough periodontal evaluation is mandatory. As part of this periodontal evaluation, each tooth should be palpated to determine the degree of tooth mobility (although by itself, tooth mobility is not the only determining factor for selecting teeth to support an overdenture). Generally, highly mobile teeth with an unfavorable crown-root ratio will become tight and firm in the alveolar ridge after coronal reduction.

Radiographic Examination

A radiograph itself is only one aid in a complete oral examination; radiographs help to determine to a certain degree the bone level and the presence of pathological conditions, which cannot be seen visually (Fig. 2-2).

Other areas of concern – such as the presence of retained roots, curvature of roots, root formation, size of roots and root canal anatomy – are some of the important things that should be evaluated.

Diagnosis

Such an examination and diagnosis helps determine which teeth can be saved to act as supporting abutments for an overlay prosthesis.

Evaluation and Selection of Abutments (for Overdentures)

When selecting abutments for support of the overdenture you should consider:

a) root form;

b) the location of the abutment;

c) amount of bone support;

d) masticatory load to be subjected against the roots;

e) amount of space between abutments;

f) how many teeth are available;

g) how many teeth are present in the opposing dentition; and

h) the preliminary design of the prosthesis.

As the overlay appliance is supported by roots, root form is an important consideration. Basically, these types may be considered:

a) flat roots;

b) conical roots;

c) curved roots; and

d) multiple-rooted teeth.

The flat roots will give good support and are very excellent candidates for overdenture abutments. Curved roots also give good support and security in the alveolar ridge, due to the locking effect of the curvature. Whenever possible, multiple-rooted teeth should be saved, particularly where there is no furcation involved. The multiple-rooted teeth give maximum support and retention for an overdenture. Conical roots are the poorest candidates as abutments for support of an overdenture.

Abutment Location

The strategic location of the abutment is very important for the support, stability and

26

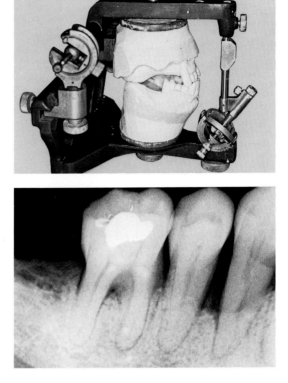

Fig. 2-1 Articulated diagnostic casts provide valuable information for more ideal diagnosis and treatment planning. The vertical space available will help to determine attachment selection. Anatomical characteristics such as tori may modify treatment and may need to be removed. Supraeruption or extrusion of teeth may require special surgical procedures to provide adequate denture space.

Fig. 2-2 Remaining bone support around the teeth is studied radiographically to aid in selecting the best roots for abutments. Roots of multi-rooted teeth can be retained as individual roots. Teeth with the most bone support and in the most strategic locations should be used as supporting abutments.

retention of the overdenture. If two are retained in one arch, the abutments are in one plane (Fig. 2-3a); if, in addition, a posterior abutment is retained, you will have abutments in two planes (Figs. 2-3b and c); now, if another abutment is retained in the opposite area, they will be in three planes. If abutments can be selected where they are located anteriorly and posteriorly (in three planes), the overdenture is provided with the greatest degree of support, stability and retention (Figs. 2-3d and e).

Bone Support

The amount of bone support around each abutment tooth is very important for the strength and support of the abutment and its preservation. Try to select the abutments with the greatest amount of bone support, particularly if they are in an ideal location for maximum stability and retention. As men-

tioned previously, root form is also important as it relates to the bone support. The greater the root surface, with its attached periodontal ligaments, the greater its supporting effect. The overdenture attachments should be placed where the abutments have the most bone support. This information and the design should always be conveyed to the dental technician.

Proximal Space Between Abutments

Space between abutments sometimes becomes an important consideration and it can be a potential problem as well. If the roots are too close, it may be impossible to design copings with wide open gingival, facial and lingual embrasure spaces for periodontal health. Eventually, periodontal problems can develop in these areas. It is often necessary to eliminate a tooth for no other reason than to produce more space between abut-

27

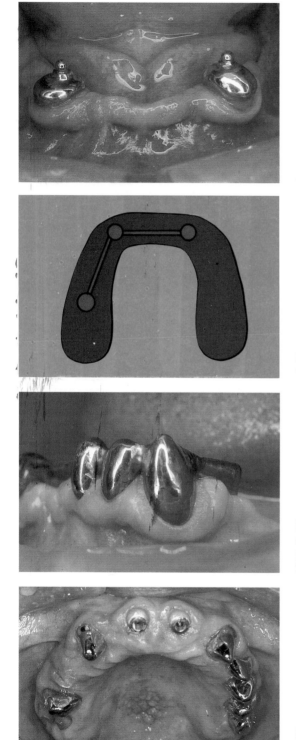

Fig. 2-3a Two cuspids in one plane is a common application in the lower arch.

Fig. 2-3b Stability in two planes is provided with two cuspids and a posterior abutment.

Fig. 2-3c Two-plane stability can also be obtained with several abutments splinted in one plane with a short single bar cantilevered distal to the strongest abutment.

Fig. 2-3d Abutments in three planes, such as these anterior and posterior abutments; provide best distribution for forces of mastication.

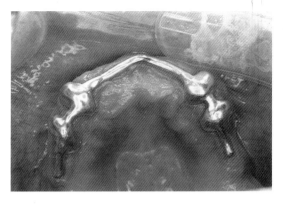

Fig. 2-3e Support in three planes provided by bar-splinted teeth, with two short bars cantilevered distally. Abutment teeth supporting short cantilevered bars must have strong bone support and only used opposite a complete denture or another overdenture.

ments. This is particularly acceptable where adequate abutments are present.

Number of Teeth Available

The greater the number of teeth available to select and retain as abutments, the better the success of the overdenture prosthesis. By saving many of these weak abutments, the forces of mastication can be shared and distributed between these abutments and the alveolar supporting structures.

Masticatory Load and the Opposing Dentition

The masticatory load imposed on the prosthesis, and, of course, the supporting structures, are important considerations. Therefore the opposing dentition must be considered too. Will the opposing dentition be a complete denture? Another overdenture? Or natural dentition? If the overdenture is to function against a complete denture or a full complement of teeth, there will be different masticatory loads transmitted to the abutment teeth and overdenture-supporting soft tissues. The opposing dentition is important when determining the number of teeth to be retained, the design of

the overlay prosthesis, the type of attachments to be used, whether the overlay prosthesis is to be tooth-supported only or a tooth-tissue supported appliance.

With a tooth-tissue supported overlay prosthesis, there is a balanced and maximum utilization of the soft tissue and abutment teeth during mastication. For example, if a lower overdenture functions against a full complement of upper teeth, the masticatory load will be heavy. Since the dentist wants to spare the roots any unnecessary load, he would design a "resilient" overlay prosthesis to maximize the amount of load transmitted to the supporting soft tissues. At the same time, the abutments help to support the overdenture during function.

Design of the Prosthesis

The design of the prosthesis should be thoroughly understood and planned before actual abutment preparation and treatment.

Is the overlay prosthesis to be supported by just plain bare roots? Are the abutments to be restored with simple copings for a telescopic overlay prosthesis? Are special attachments to be incorporated to improve retention and stability of the removable prosthesis? These are just a few of the things to be considered.

Chapter 3

Treatment Planning

Treatment of Multiple Problems

Probably one of the most challenging, perplexing and difficult phases of overdenture prosthetics is developing a treatment plan for the various oral conditions present.

Since most overdenture patients are terminal cases dentally, a complexity of problems may be present. There may be advanced periodontal disease, with some teeth so hopelessly involved that periodontal therapy would be difficult without removing these hopeless teeth first.

The teeth to be saved may have minimal bone support, so that they have to be reduced to produce a more favorable crown-root ratio. This makes endodontics mandatory. Removal or reduction of teeth poses an esthetic problem. The patient needs some form of temporary prosthesis to be worn during the treatment and healing phase. Furthermore, there may be surgical problems that must be corrected first.

All of these procedures require careful coordination with the various specialists, if such are utilized, including coordination with the dental laboratory. Finally, each patient should be treated in the most efficient and comfortable manner possible.

Coordination of Multiple Treatments

When developing your treatment plan you must consider the following:

Will Special Surgical Procedures or Extractions be Necessary?

1. Will the useless teeth be extracted before periodontal surgery?
2. Can these extractions be made after periodontal surgery?
3. Can the extractions be made during periodontal surgery?

Will Periodontal Surgery be Necessary?

1. Will periodontal surgery be performed first?
2. Can periodontal therapy be completed without extracting the useless teeth?
3. Must periodontal surgery be performed after extractions because of the involved periodontal condition of the neighboring hopeless teeth?
4. Can an interim overdenture be used as the periodontal dressing if the teeth are reduced prior to periodontal surgery?
5. Must the interim overdenture be worn during periodontal healing?

Will Endodontics be Necessary?

1. Will endodontics be completed before reduction of clinical crowns?
2. Will endodontics be finished when the clinical crowns are reduced?
3. Will endodontics be finished at some date after reduction of clinical crowns?

Will an Interim Overdenture be Necessary?

1. Will the reduction of the clinical crowns require an interim overdenture to meet the patient's demands for comfort, function and cosmetics?
2. Will the interim appliance be customized from an existing prosthesis?
3. Will it be fabricated similar to an immediate complete denture?
4. Will the interim overdenture be used as the final overdenture?

Various Categories of Patients with Multiple Dental Problems

Overdenture patients generally fall into certain categories of dental problems. Identifying the best possible sequence of treatments for each specific condition works to the benefit of the patient and dentist.

Overdenture Condition I

The treatment plan associated with this category is the simplest to manage.

1. Neither periodontal disease is present nor is extensive treatment required.
2. The remaining teeth have adequate bone support and do not need to be reduced to make a more favorable crown-root ratio. Preparations for long copings are made.
3. Therefore, no endodontics is necessary.
4. No extractions are necessary.
5. No special interim overdenture is necessary. Generally, the patient has an existing prosthesis that can be modified around the temporary crowns placed on the prepared abutments.

In this situation, therefore, there is no necessity for periodontics, endodontics or extractions. Any periodontal problem that may be present can be treated with simple soft tissue curettage and root planing procedures. Endodontics is not necessary, because the abutment crown-root ratio is favorable with good bone support. As no extractions are required, there is no need for the replacement of missing teeth with another removable prosthesis. Such patients are generally wearing some type of removable prosthesis.

Treatment Plan Sequence

This situation is the simplest for management and treatment planning. After tooth preparation, temporary crowns are placed on the abutments and fitted to the existing prosthesis. This modified prosthesis is worn until the final prosthesis is completed and inserted.

Overdenture Condition II

The following treatment sequence is somewhat similar to that of Condition I with the exception of periodontal therapy and the possible need for extractions. In this situation, periodontal therapy will be necessary, and there is no esthetic problem requiring an interim overdenture before the operative appointments. Briefly:

1. There is periodontal disease which has to be treated before the first operative appointment.
2. Extractions may be required.
3. However, extractions pose no esthetic problem, so the patient will not require an initial interim prosthesis.
4. However, an interim overdenture may be necessary during operative therapy if the teeth are reduced.
5. Endodontics may be necessary if the teeth are reduced.

When periodontal therapy or extractions are necessary – and there is no immediate esthetic problem – the same procedure is followed as with Condition I, with a slight variation.

Suppose the patient has all or most of his maxillary dentition and involved with advanced periodontal disease. The posteriors which are hopeless, need to be extracted and the anteriors retained. Generally, the patient will not need an immediate temporary prosthesis.

Treatment Plan Sequence

The patient is treated in this manner: First, the hopeless posterior teeth are removed (this is similar to the treatment of a complete denture patient, when the posterior ridges are allowed to heal before removal of the anterior teeth and insertion of the complete denture). The periodontal therapy is then performed on the retained anterior teeth, and the tissue is permitted to heal and mature for two to three months. Only after tissue maturation should the teeth be prepared and a temporary prosthesis provided. Consequently, this interim overdenture is needed only if the anterior teeth are reduced to create a favorable crown-root ratio – and even then, it will be worn for only a short time. Endodontics may be necessary but can be performed at any time, preferably after tooth reduction.

Overdenture Condition III

This situation requires the maximum coordination of all phases of treatment. Unfortunately, it is the condition found in most candidates for overdenture treatment. You may expect to find:

1. Some teeth with no bone support must be removed to facilitate periodontal therapy.
2. Periodontal surgery is necessary.

3. Generally, extractions must be performed prior to periodontal surgery for more effective periodontal therapy.
4. Endodontics is generally necessary.
5. There will be an esthetic problem since anterior teeth are removed.
6. Thus, an interim overdenture will be required due to the location of the extractions and reduction of clinical crowns.

This type of dental situation will be considered in much more detail. It is one of those most commonly treated. Often, one will observe a patient suffering extensive multiple dental problems. There is advanced periodontal disease with extensive bone loss around some of the teeth to be retained. Other teeth may have no bone support and must be removed first, in order to treat the other teeth periodontially. Removal of these teeth presents a patient management problem, since some form of transitional prosthetic replacement must be provided to enable the patient to function with satisfactory cosmetics during healing. Since the teeth to be retained have minimal bone support, they must be reduced to produce a more favorable crown-root ratio. Of course, reduction of such teeth makes endodontics mandatory; this can be performed before, during or after the extractions and periodontal surgery.

The dentist's immediate concern should be to get the patient comfortable and under complete management and control as rapidly as possible. This is accomplished rapidly by reducing the height of the clinical crowns to the alveolar ridge (if maximum favorable crown-root ratio is desired); perform or complete endodontics; extract the hopeless teeth; complete periodontal surgery; and insert an interim overdenture. In this manner, the patient is provided comfort, function and cosmetics, rapidly.

With this in mind, the authors recommend the following procedure as the fastest and simplest approach.

Treatment Plan Sequence

Outline of the Clinical Phase	Outline of the Laboratory Phase
1. Examination, Diagnosis and Treatment Plan:	
a) Patient history.	
b) Clinical examination.	
c) Radiographs.	
d) Impressions for study casts (to be used for articulated fabrication of interim overdenture and to determine attachment selection.	1. Impressions poured for study casts. 2. Casts articulated. 3. Interim overdenture fabrication.
2. Prophylaxis, soft tissue curettage, root planing, home care instructions.	
3. Operative Appointment No. 1 (long appointment; this is the extensive treatment stage):	
a) Reduce abutment teeth to 1-2 millimeters (mm) above gingiva for short copings; longer preparations for longer copings.	
b) Initial endodontics or complete endodontics at one sitting.	
c) Extract all hopeless teeth or individual roots of multiple-rooted teeth.	
d) Complete periodontal surgery.	
e) Insert interim overdenture.	1. Completed earlier.
4. Operative Appointment No. 2 (after initial healing of several weeks):	
a) Complete endodontics (if not completed).	
b) Impressions for casts to produce custom impression trays for master impression.	2. Casts for fabrication of custom impression trays. 3. Custom impression trays.
5. Operative Appointment No. 3 (after complete surgical healing and maturation of tissue; 2-3 months. Longer for multiple extractions; 4-6 months –?):	
a) Final abutment preparation.	
b) Impressions of abutments for master working cast for copings.	3. a) Master cast with removable dies. b) Coping fabrication. c) Attachments placed on copings.

Treatment Plan Sequence

Outline of the Clinical Phase	Outline of the Laboratory Phase

6. Operative Appointment No. 4
  a) Try-in of castings
    (castings should have attachments).
  b) Master impression of denture supporting areas and of abutments with castings in place (for fabrication of overdenture).
	4. a) Master cast with copings in place for fabrication of overlay prosthesis.
	  b) Occlusal registration trays with occlusal rims.

7. Operative Appointment No. 5
  a) Occlusal registration.
	5. a) Casts articulated.
	  b) Denture teeth set-up.

8. Operative Appointment No. 6 a) Check trial set-up of teeth for esthetics. Remount occlusal records.	6. Occlusal refinement. 7. Overdenture processed.

9. Operative Appointment No. 7
  a) Cementation of substructure and insertion of overlay prosthesis.
  b) Home care instructions for dental disease control, nutrition, and maintenance of substructure and overdenture.	

Though you may be able to reduce the number of steps, be careful that the shortcuts do not affect the success of the final prosthesis. For example; the initial master impression taken of the abutment teeth and tissue-bearing mucosa (that will be used to produce a master cast for coping fabrication) can also serve as the master cast for the overdenture construction. However, the author strongly advise against this procedure. Sawing and trimming the dies will destroy the accuracy and usefulness of this original cast for fabrication of a quality overdenture. Expansion and clarification of the Outline.

Now, let us discuss in more detail each of the steps outlined above.

Examination

A thorough clinical and radiographic examination with accurately articulated study casts is the most important initial step. The study casts are then used by the laboratory technician to fabricate an interim overdenture. This appliance will thus be available during the initial operative phase of treatment.

Prophylaxis

Before any periodontal surgery is performed, the general health of the tissues should be improved by soft tissue curettage and root planing. However, this may be a problem when teeth to be extracted have extensive periodontal disease with granulation tissue completely surrounding these teeth. In a situation like this, it is usually best to thoroughly curette only the abutment teeth and the gross calculus deposits from the teeth indicated for extraction. The balance of the diseased tissue can be removed with the extraction of the teeth.

Remember, the overdenture patient has neglected his oral hygiene for years. You should begin instruction in brushing, flossing, etc. Now – before proceeding with active treatment, since bad habits are hard to break. Repeat the instructions frequently even after the overdenture is inserted, before the substructure is inserted and frequently thereafter.

Operative Appointment No. 1

This initial operative appointment is generally the longest, when most of the extensive dental procedures are initiated or completed. During this appointment the rather complicated dental problems can be reduced to easily manageable tasks. The single most important item making this possible is the interim overdenture. During this visit the patient should come under complete management.

Root Reduction

The first step is to reduce the abutment teeth to the approximate height for their coping types (Fig. 3-1). The dentist must have a mental image of the coping height, with the understanding that after periodontal healing additional abutment reduction may be necessary. The coping heights determining abutment reduction are:

a) Short copings – 1-2mm above gingiva (Fig. 3-2).
b) Medium-short copings – 3-4mm above gingiva (Fig. 3-3).

c) Medium copings – 4-6mm above gingiva (Fig. 3-4).
d) Long copings – 6-8mm above gingiva (Fig. 3-5).

When long copings are to be used, the teeth are not devitalized and the maximum occlusal reduction is done using the pulp location as the guide. Remember, do not expose the pulp tissue. However, with adults this reduction can be substantial, since often there is extensive pulpal recession. When there is pulpal recession in adults, the abutments may be reduced for medium copings without exposing the pulp tissue. Generally, pulp exposure is certain for the shorter preparations, thus requiring endodontics.

Remember, the abutments will be longer after periodontal surgery and healing. They must be reduced accordingly when the final preparations are made. These coping types and preparations are determined in part by the amount of supporting bone remaining. The specific forms of copings will be discussed in greater detail in the chapter on "Preparations." Since overdenture patients generally have severe periodontal problems with extensive bone loss, short copings are indicated.

Lastly, after the initial occlusal reduction, semi-prepare the abutments by removing gross undercuts to give the abutments a slight tapering form for retention of the interim overdenture (Fig. 3-6). This shaping is done after endodontic therapy and the sealing of the canal with a temporary stopping.

Endodontic Therapy

When only a few teeth require endodontics, it is just as convenient to complete this procedure earlier. When multiple endodontics is necessary, therapy can be simplified and reduced to a very easy and simple procedure by the elimination of the clinical crown first. (See a simplified approach to Endodontics," chapter 5.) The general practitioner must decide if he will perform this

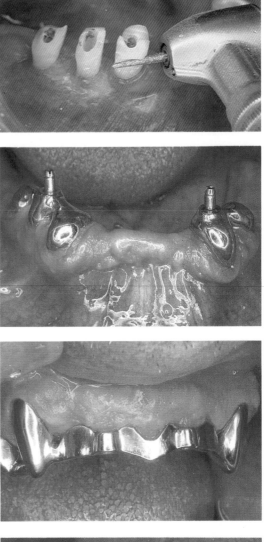

Fig. 3-1 Initial reduction of abutments is made by sectioning through the clinical crowns with a fissure bur. The level of this initial cut is determined by the approximate height of the coping type. Further reduction and modification may be necessary after periodontal surgery and healing.

Fig. 3-2 Short coping used with a stud attachment. Short copings extend 1-2 millimeters above the gingiva and conform closely to the contour of the alveolar ridge.

Fig. 3-3 Medium-short copings splinted together and used with a connecting bar attachment. These copings are slightly longer (3-4 millimeters above the gingiva) than short copings. Such copings, when splinted, have more room for developing ideal gingival, facial and lingual embrasures than with very short copings.

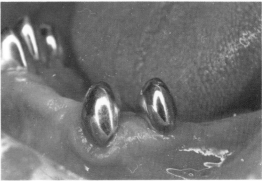

Fig. 3-4 Medium copings (4-6 millimeters) provide support, stability and retention for an overdenture. These copings may be designed to provide only support and stability, or also retention.

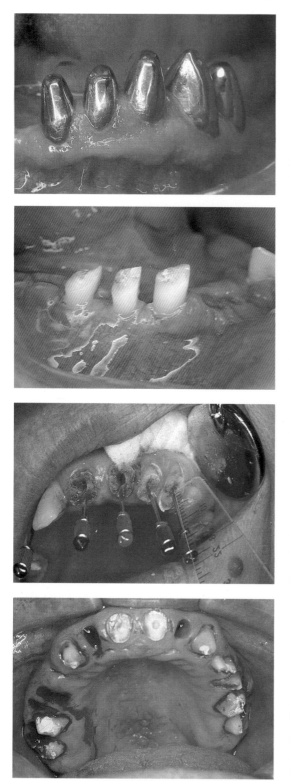

Fig. 3-5 Long copings (6-8 millimeters long) being used to support a telescopic overdenture. The form and taper will determine its function. A tapered form provides primarily, support and stability. When portions of the proximal walls are parallel, retention is possible.

Fig. 3-6 Abutments "rough-prepared" by reducing the gross undercuts. These semi-prepared abutments help to retain the interim overdenture after periodontal healing and during tissue maturation.

Fig. 3-7 Endodontics is initiated or completed through the shortened teeth. If only initial treatment is performed, each root can be instrumented up to a 30-35 reamer, treated with a medicament, a small ball of cotton moistened with the medicament placed in the top of the portion of the canal and the canal opening filled with a cement stopping. Endodontics is completed more leisurely later. When many roots are retained this is the treatment of choice. Or, endodontics can be completed now when fewer abutments are treated.

Fig. 3-8 Hopeless teeth with inadequate bone support are removed. Questionable roots of multiple-rooted teeth are generally removed during periodontal surgery. The removal of these hopeless teeth makes it possible to eliminate all of the diseased tissue and infection that would interfere with periodontal surgery.

comparatively easy and simple procedure, or refer the patient to an endodontist.

If the latter is the elected approach, after tooth reduction, instrument each canal using tactile sensation for instrument length control. Instrument the canals to a 30 to 35 reamer (Fig. 3-7); treat and seal in a medicament with a temporary stopping similar to standard endodontic procedures. The patient then can be referred to the endodontist for completion of treatment at some later date. Since in this case this procedure will be performed by a specialist, of course it would be to the general practitioner's benefit to have these teeth treated endodontically first. Then he need not be concerned with this initial endodontic therapy when the crowns are removed. However, when many teeth are involved it is kinder to the patient to have this time-consuming and tedious procedure performed on root stubs rather than the whole tooth.

When the general practitioner elects to perform this simple task, as the author recommend, it may be accomplished in one of several ways.

For example:

1. *Initial treatment performed immediately after crown reduction*

   a) Reduce the crown.
   b) Enlarge the canal opening with a No. 4 round bur approximately 4 mm deep. This provides space for a cotton pledget and temporary stopping.
   c) Rapidly instrument the canal to a 30-35 reamer and file. Use tactile sensation to instrument short of the apex.
   d) Treat the canal with a medicament.
   e) Seal a cotton pledget with medicament into the canal opening and seal the opening with a temporary stopping.

Root canal therapy can then be finished later according to the dentist's and patient's convenience, during the healing phase after periodontal surgery.

2. *Endodontic therapy completed*

   Immediately after the crowns are reduced, root canal therapy can be initiated and completed. Use the rapid, simplified and conventional technique discussed in the chapter on "Endodontic Therapy."

Extractions

All hopeless teeth should be removed at this time. Roots of multi-rooted teeth can be eliminated during periodontal therapy, when a more definite diagnosis of the prognosis of these roots can be ascertained (Fig. 3-8).

Periodontal Surgery

As with endodontics, often periodontal surgery is best performed after extractions. It is often impossible to periodontally treat these abutment teeth near teeth with extensively diseased granulation tissue completely surrounding them. Removal of these hopeless teeth is necessary in order to more effectively perform periodontal surgery on the retained abutments. But it is this single fact that requires a coordinated treatment plan if these procedures are to be shared with several dentists. It is always kinder to the patient to combine extractions and periodontal treatment (Fig. 3-9). These surgical procedures should not be separated simply for the convenience of the dentists, but only if better results can be expected. Treatment is tremendously simplified if the dentist either performs all procedures himself, or works in close harmony with the periodontist.

There are several ways to manage periodontal therapy:

a) All periodontal therapy performed by the specialist or general dentist before abutment preparations.

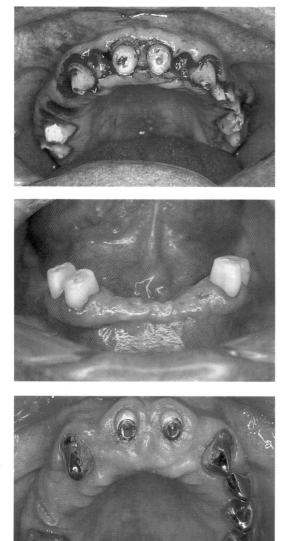

Fig. 3-9 Periodontal therapy is completed after tooth reduction and extractions of hopeless teeth. Reduction of the clinical crowns and removal of all hopeless roots and teeth simplifies periodontal therapy by providing better access.

Fig. 3-10 The previously "rough-prepared" abutments now extend substantially above the healed gingival tissues. These abutments must now be prepared for the selected coping type.

Fig. 3-11 Finished copings cemented on the abutments prior to taking a muscle-trimmed impression for the overdenture. When the copings are cemented in place, a master cast is produced of the alveolar ridges and copings. The copings are not cemented if they are to be "pulled with the impression to become an integral part of the master cast."

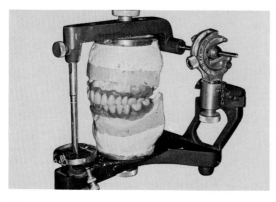

Fig. 3-12 The denture set-up completed and should be checked in the mouth for accurate intraocclusal records and esthetics. The position of the anterior teeth can be changed at chairside for a more natural appearance. This, in itself, is a very important factor for patient acceptance.

b) All treatment by the general dentist during the initial operative appointment: reduction of clinical crowns, endodontics (initial or completed), extractions, periodontal therapy and interim overdenture insertion.

c) Treatment shared by the general dentist and periodontist: here the general dentist reduces the crowns, performs endodontics (initial only), extractions, and the specialist completes periodontal therapy and fits the interim overdenture.

The closer the two doctors work together, the less trauma for the patient. Ideally, the dentists should use a team approach, performing all procedures in one office.
Here is a suggested general dentist-specialist team approach to overdenture-periodontal therapy if periodontal surgery was not completed earlier.

General practitioner:

a) Prepared interim overdenture is available for use.
b) Rapidly reduce all teeth.
c) Perform only initial endodontic therapy when there are numerous teeth to be treated.
d) Semi-prepare the abutments.
e) Extract all hopeless teeth.
f) Fit interim overdenture over the abutments.

Specialist:

a) Periodontal surgery in same office, immediately.
b) Patient transferred to nearby specialist for immediate treatment.
c) The patient is dismissed for periodontal surgery at a later date.

When periodontal surgery is to be performed by the periodontist (following the philosophy of least trauma for the patient's convenience and comfort) professional cooperation can be difficult. Often, the offices of the specialist and generalist are miles apart and any form of team effort is difficult or impossible. In such situations, often it is necessary to have the periodontal therapy completed later after the healing of the extraction sites. Often this is desirable to allow time for the filling-in of bone prior to periodontal therapy. Each practitioner must work out the overall best arrangement considering the patient's well-being, comfort and results.

Operative Appointment No. 2
(after initial healing; two to three weeks)

a) Completion of endodontics. If this treatment was not completed initially, utilize standard endodontic procedure to complete all endodontics (See "A Simplified Approach to Endodontics," chapter 5).
b) Impression for custom impression tray. Accurate alginate impressions should be made to form casts for construction of custom trays for impressions of prepared abutments later.

Operative Appointment No. 3

Make final abutment preparations only after healing and maturation of the tissues. Depending upon the extensiveness of extractions and periodontal therapy, a minimum of 2-8 months should be allowed for this healing. When numerous teeth are extracted, healing and maturation of the edentulous areas should be permitted for a much longer time – 8-10 months. However, 2-3 months appears to be sufficient time for periodontal tissue maturation.

Abutment Preparations

These are made according to the coping types selected. You will notice that after periodontal surgery and healing, the abutments now extend farther above the gingiva than at original reduction (Fig. 3-10).

Impressions

Where multiple abutments are prepared, it is advisable to take a master impression of the abutments only for coping fabrication and attachment processing. Single impressions with compound and copper bands may be taken of the individual abutments.

It is important to remember that an impression for the overdenture prosthesis must accurately record the denture-bearing mucosa, preferably muscle-trimmed. Taking an impression of the abutments while muscle-trimming often leads to an inaccurate impression. In addition, cutting and trimming the dies essentially destroys the master cast for fabrication of a quality overdenture. Thus, it is best to take a second impression later for the overdenture proper, with the castings fitted in place. The impression is poured then with appropriate stone materials to construct a cast with removable dies.

Operative Appointment No. 4

Try-in of the Castings

With their attachments installed, the try-in eliminates one of the most common problems with the fit of the overdenture prosthesis. Test the fit of each coping on its abutment to detect any errors in the impression; or inaccuracies in the laboratory phase of coping fabrication: splinting, soldering, or attachment assembly. Using this approach, if problems later arise when inserting the overdenture over the cemented substructure, you can concentrate on the overdenture when looking for the problem rather than the fit of the substructure on the abutments.

Master Overdenture Impressions

With the castings in place, an accurate muscle-trimmed impression is possible (Fig.

3-11). The castings can be withdrawn with the impression; or, the castings can be cemented. Cementation does eliminate any question in the fit of the prosthesis due to errors accompanying cementation. With some attachments, special procedures must be followed when an impression is taken of the alveolar ridges and abutments with copings cemented. This is necessary as stone reproductions of the attachment may not be strong enough to withstand the manipulation of overdenture fabrication. In such situations, for example, with many stud attachments, it may be necessary to utilize transfer males (this technique will be covered in great detail later in this text); or duplicate the attachment portion in a hard apoxy die material. If you have not cemented the coping, it is often best to withdraw the coping substructure with the impression and then pour in stone to form a master cast. Thus the copings and their attachments become an integral part of the cast during overdenture fabrication.

Operative Appointment No. 5

Occlusal Registration

Accurate occlusal records should be obtained using custom record bases made on the master cast. Use the technique of your choice for taking these records: intraoral tracers, customized trays with occlusal record rims, or even with the metal overdenture framework with the female portion of the attachments secured to the framework, can be snapped over the substructure to make an abutment-supported and retained occlusal registration.

Operative Appointment No. 6

A trial set-up of the denture teeth can be approved by the patient for shade, mold and natural arrangement. The occlusal relationship of the denture teeth can be evaluated for centric as well as for all functional movements. The overdenture is now ready for completion in the laboratory (Fig. 3-12).

Operative Appointment No. 7

Cementation

Cement the substructure, if you did not cement it during operative appointment No. 4 (Fig. 3-11). Insert the overdenture. Give the patient complete instructions in the use and function of the prosthesis.

Home Care Instructions

No overdenture technique is complete without thorough and frequent instruction in dental home care. This should include instruction in proper toothbrushing technique, use of dental floss, as well as the use of fluoride and other special aids. Include counseling on proper diet and nutrition.

Chapter 4

Abutment and Coping Considerations

General Abutment Consideration

Abutments should be selected only after a complete and thorough examination as discussed earlier. Criteria for selection include:

1. Location of abutments: try to select abutments in more than one plane for maximum support and stability.
2. Bone support: select abutments with the most bone support for maximum strength.
3. Root form: flat, curved and multi-rooted teeth make better abutments than short conical roots.
4. Space between abutments: inadequate space between very close roots may make satisfactory embrasure form between copings difficult.
5. Number of teeth available: often the selection of ideal abutments will be determined by the number of teeth available.
6. Masticatory load – opposing dentition: whether the opposing dentition is normal dentition, another overdenture, or a complete denture will help to determine the chewing forces present. Differences in the strength of the muscles of mastication vary from patient to patient – this must be taken into consideration when selecting abutments.
7. Design of prosthesis: the design of the prosthesis is normally determined in part by the abutments present and their location rather than selecting abutments based upon the type of appliance. How-

ever, often abutments (when available to select from) may be selected on the basis of the attachment selection planned.

Coping Types

A coping fitted to a prepared abutment is called a primary coping. The sleeve, or coping, that fits over this primary coping is referred to as a secondary coping.

There are four basic types of primary copings:

1. Long copings (6-8 mm).
2. Medium copings (4-6 mm).
3. Medium-short copings (2-4 mm).
4. Short copings (1-2 mm).

Which coping is best for a specific abutment depends on the amount of alveolar support, whether or not the abutment is vital, and the function of the coping and overlay prosthesis.

Long Copings
(6-8 millimeters for vital teeth)

The long coping is an excellent restoration, applicable to many overlay techniques (Fig. 4-1a). It may be used simply to provide stability and retention under a telescopic overdenture, or retention may be improved by combining the coping with a small plunger-like attachment that engages a small round depression cut into the proximal surface (Fig. 4-1b). Long copings may also be splint-

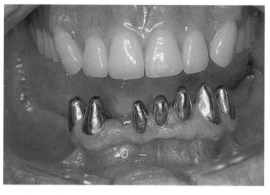

Fig. 4-1a Multiple abutments restored with long copings designed to support and retain a telescopic overdenture. Long copings are generally used with vital teeth having adequate bone support.

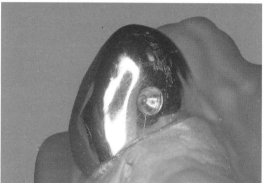

Fig. 4-1b Long coping with a small round depression that will be engaged by the plunger of an IC attachment (a springloaded plunger attachment).

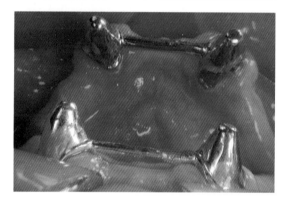

Fig. 4-1c Long copings splinted with a bar. The bar provides the retention for the overdenture. These long copings are very tapered in form. Parallelism of coping walls is not necessary as retention is obtained with the bar attachment.

ed with special bar-like attachments (Fig. 4-1c).

There are two types of long copings, depending on the form of the coping and how it is to function with the overlay prosthesis.

1. If the long primary coping fits inside the resin denture base of the overlay prosthesis, the resin denture base acts as the secondary coping. The long primary coping should have a general tapering form tapered heavily on the facial surface to allow room for denture tooth set up; less heavily on the lingual surface (Fig. 4-2a). The gingival one-half to one-third of the proximal surfaces should be approximately parallel to each other and to the proximal surfaces of the other abutment cop-

Figs. 4-2a to c   Long copings (6-8 millimeters long):

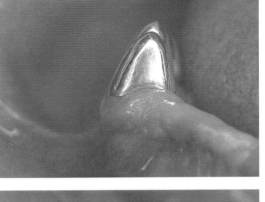

Fig. 4-2a   Proximal view of a long coping showing its tapering form. It should be tapered more from the facial and toward the lingual to provide maximum room for the set-up of the anterior denture teeth. Therefore maximum facial reduction of the abutment is important.

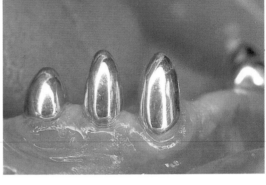

Fig. 4-2b   Facial view of a long coping designed for retention for a telescopic overdenture. The gingival one-third to one-half of the proximal surfaces are approximately parallel to each other. The occlusal one-half to two-thirds of the proximal surfaces are tapering.

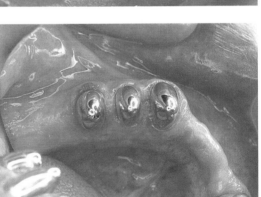

Fig. 4-2c   Occlusal view of copings showing a tapering form. Notice that the absence of crown contours provides maximum tissue exposure and overdenture tissue contact.

ings. The occlusal one-third to one-half of these proximal surfaces should be very tapered (Figs. 4-2b and c).

There should be no gingival bulges to the contour of the coping. Otherwise, space will be present below this height of contour gingivally and between the tissue surface of the overlay prosthesis. In such a situation, there will be an unhealthy pro-liferation of gingival tissues into this space.

2. If a metal or porcelain-to-metal secondary coping is to fit over the primary coping, the long primary coping must have a heavy shoulder at the gingival margin (Fig. 4-3).

The coping should taper gradually on all surfaces but more heavily on the facial

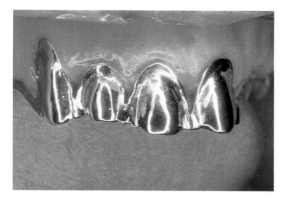

Fig. 4-3 Primary copings designed to receive porcelain-to-metal secondary copings. Note the definite shoulder located just at the crest of the gingiva. The gingival portion of the secondary coping fits snugly against this shoulder. If frictional resistance between the primary and secondary copings is to retain the overdenture, the overall contour of the primary coping is similar to that shown in Fig. 4-2b. The contour of the coping is very tapered when auxiliary retention for the overdenture is used. Adjacent copings are splinted near the incisal with well-developed interproximal spaces. These gingival, facial and lingual embrasures are very important for periodontal health.

surface. No parallel proximal walls are necessary, since this coping design is generally used in conjunction with some form of auxiliary attachment such as a bar. However, if a plunger-type of auxiliary attachment is to be used, one flattened proximal area will be necessary to receive a round depression engaged by the plunger.

Medium Copings
(4-6 millimeters for vital and non-vital teeth)

Medium-sized copings may be used with vital teeth where the pulp has receded or with non-vital teeth having adequate bone support. Medium-sized copings are not generally designed as individual copings for retention of the overlay prosthesis due to parallel coping walls (Fig. 4-4a). They are generally connected with some type of bar attachment. Or, they may also be used with auxiliary plunger or pressure-button attachments. They are conical with greater taper on all surfaces, particularly the facial surface when used with bar attachments (Fig. 4-4b). If used with a plunger-button attachment, the surface engaged by the plunger is flattened.

Medium-Short Copings
(2-4 millimeters for non-vital teeth)

Medium-short copings are indicated for non-vital teeth, where a more favorable crown-root ratio is desired than that possible with medium or long copings (Fig. 4-5). This coping form (and preparation) is indicated when: it is difficult to obtain auxiliary retention of the coping on the abutment with a dowel or parallel pins (the proximal walls of the preparation should be very closely parallel for maximum frictional fit of the coping); numerous neighboring abutments are to be splinted, thus permitting better embrasure formation than possible with very short copings; used with bar attachments.

Short Copings
(1-2 millimeters for non-vital teeth)

Short copings are fabricated to conform to the curvature of the alveolar ridge, with a very low profile. They are indicated for maximum favorable crown-root ratio (Fig. 4-6). Such short copings are particularly suited to various types of stud attachments, but may also be used effectively with many forms of bar attachments. These coping forms will be discussed in more detail later.

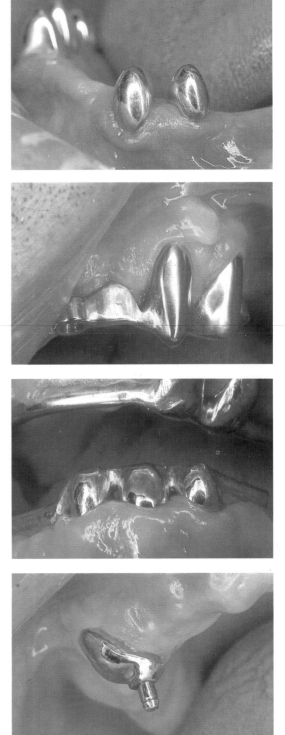

Fig. 4-4a Medium copings (4-6 millimeters long): They are approximately 4-6 millimeters long and provide support and stability but no retention here.

Fig. 4-4b Medium copings connected with a bar for retention. The general contour is tapering, designed to occupy minimal space and provide a favorable crown-root ratio.

Fig. 4-5 Medium-short copings (3-4 millimeters long): Multiple medium-short copings splinted together and connected to a bar for auxiliary retention. The slightly parallel proximal root preparation provides some retention for the coping. Note the well-developed gingival embrasures for periodontal health.

Fig. 4-6 Short copings (1-2 millimeters long): A short coping fitted with a stud attachment (Gerber). The contour is convex and conforms closely to the form of the alveolar ridge to provide maximum room for anterior teeth. Such an arrangement decreases the crown-root ratio and allows maximum room for the denture teeth. This is an important consideration when making short abutment preparations.

The Relation of Coping Type to Alveolar Support and Vitality

When one-half or less of the abutment root is supported by bone, the crown should be reduced to provide the most favorable crown – root ratio, particularly if only a few abutments remain. Such roots may be prepared to receive short or medium-short copings. The teeth will be non-vital, having been treated endodontically. However, if there is adequate alveolar support (one-half or more of the root length), improving the crown-root ratio may not be as critical, particularly if the opposing dentition is not natural dentition. Here the dentist may choose to leave the abutments vital, and thus eliminate the need for endodontics. Now medium copings (if there is pulpal recession) or long copings may be indicated. Table A summarizes the relationship of coping design to alveolar bone support and tooth vitality.

Table A:
Coping Form and Portion of Root Supported by Bone

	½ or less	½	½ or more
Vital		Medium Copings (where pulp receded)	Medium Copings Long Copings
Non-Vital	Short Copings Med.-Short Copings	Medium Copings Med.-Short Copings Short Copings	Medium Copings Med.-Short Copings Short Copings

Chapter 5

Endodontics

When advanced peridontal disease has destroyed much of the supporting structure, teeth become unstable, with an unfavorable crown-root ratio (Fig. 5-1). A more favorable crown-root ratio is imperative for long-term retention of these teeth. Such teeth may be reduced to provide this favorable crown-root ratio when they can then successfully function as overdenture abutments. Such reduction of clinical crowns generally makes root canal therapy mandatory.

Often the teeth have vital pulps and endodontic therapy can be completed in one visit. Most overdenture patients also have multiple problems, requiring periodontal therapy and extractions as well as endodontics. It is often difficult to determine whether endodontics should be done before, during, or after the initial operative appointment.

Endodontics Before Operative Appointment

When only a few teeth remain, root canal therapy can best be performed on these teeth prior to abutment preparation. Then, when the teeth are reduced during the operative appointment, one does not need to be concerned with root canal therapy. This will simplify this very busy first operative appointment.

Endodontics during Initial Operative Appointment

This time-consuming, meticulous procedure can be reduced to a simplified procedure, requiring just a fraction of the time necessary for customary root canal procedures. Of course, the object of the root canal therapy is the aseptic instrumentation of the root canal space to accept a positive seal by an acceptable sealer. The more rapidly and simply that this procedure can be performed, the more efficiently the patient's problems can be managed.

But what can make endodontics a time-consuming procedure? This is normally due to difficult access, a constant need for accurate instrumentation of the canal, loss of time waiting for frequent radiographs to determine instrument position, and working on one tooth at a time. Many of these problems can be simplified by eliminating the clinical crown for better access and length control and by rapid film developing processes. This can be accomplished easily and rapidly in the following manner; 1. remove the clinical crown for direct access to the canal; 2. treat many roots at one time; 3. mechanized instrumentation; 4. special techniques for accurate length control; 5. controlled obturation; and 6. rapid radiograph processing. For example:

Providing Access

Providing access with direct vision for instrumentation is probably the single most impor-

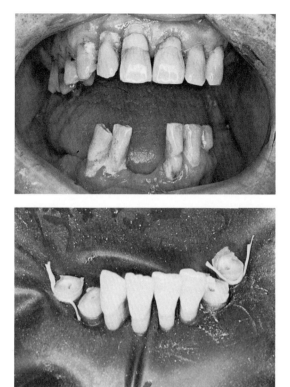

Fig. 5-1 Advanced periodontal disease has caused extreme bone loss and teeth with unfavorable crown-root ratios. Such teeth must be treated endodontically and reduced in length to control some of the destructive lateral forces. Weak and mobile teeth soon become stable and firm in their sockets after reduction.

Fig. 5-2 Teeth isolated with a rubber dam reduced to 2-4 millimeters above the gingiva (depending upon coping height). A carbide fissure bur such as the 557 was used to cut rapidly through each root. Elimination of the clinical crown improves access for root canal instrumentation.

tant procedure for more accurate and efficient root canal therapy. Since the clinical crowns will be eliminated eventually to make a favorable crown-root ratio, why not reduce the clinical crowns of all the abutment teeth prior to root canal therapy (Fig. 5-2). Such direct access reduces a procedure normally requiring an hour or more to a simple 15-20 minute technique. Often 3 to 4 teeth can be treated in a single hour. In addition, the elimination of the clinical crown will often change a previously curved tooth to a straight root tip, making instrumentation easier.

In conventional root canal therapy, the operator makes the smallest possible hole in the crown so as not to destroy it. This is not necessary for overdenture abutments. A much larger access hole can be made in the crowns of teeth to improve direct visability and entrance into the canal openings. As the clinical crowns will eventually be eliminated, this larger access hole is insignificant.

Treating Many Roots at One Time

Rather than treat one tooth at a time, all retained roots in one arch should be treated at the same time. It is just as convenient to treat 3, 4, 5, etc., roots at one time, as it is to complete each root individually.

If numerous teeth are scheduled for endodontics, the patient probably requires treatment more involved than simple crown reduction. There may be scheduled extractions, periodontal surgery and insertion of an interim overdenture. Therefore, the immediate need may be the reduction of the clinical crowns, elimination of the hopeless teeth, periodontal surgery, as well as insertion of the interim overdenture for healing, and the satisfactory management of the patient. Now the operator may wish to briefly instrument the canal to remove all pulpal tissue and then seal in a medicament with a temporary stopping. Now completion of root canal therapy can be performed more leisurely later for the convenience and comfort of the patient and dentist. Or, the patient can be referred to an endodontist for finalization of therapy.

Instrumentation and Length Control

Since successful endodontics requires that instrumentation be thorough and confined to the canal, an accurate technique for length control for instrumentation is absolutely necessary. Forcing debris or bacteria beyond the apex will cause inflammation or even infection, so length control must be maintained at all times.

Length control techniques may use some of the following:

1. Radiographic length of the roots.
2. Radiographic length of an instrument placed in the canal; then measuring from the incisal edge of the tooth to the hub of the instrument.
3. Using a special millimeter grid[1] with a radiographic pin target[2].

Dentists are familiar with the first two length control procedures; however, the third (and least known) is particularly applicable to overdenture abutments.

Pin-Grid Length Control Instrumentation Technique

Accurate root length measurement is one of the exacting requirements for satisfactory endodontics. When treating many teeth at one time, this can be solved by a technique

[1] Medidenta, Woodside, N.Y.
[2] Whaledent International, New York, N.Y.

the authors refer to as the 'pin-grid technique.' The primary object is to rapidly record all root lengths in millimeters from the apex of each root to its cut surface.

It is accomplished in this manner: a flat-headed pin is inserted into the canal opening so that its flat head rests on the cut root surface. Now a radiograph is made with a periapical film taped to a special millimeter grid. The metal grid is then superimposed on the radiograph, automatically recording the length of the root in millimeters.

The following materials are necessary to accurately measure the length of the root using this radiographic technique:

1. Flat-headed pins (use a platinum iridium pin from the parallel pin technique) (Fig. 5-3a).
2. A millimeter grid (Fig. 5-3b).

Procedure for Rapid Endodontics

1. Isolate all teeth to be treated with a rubber dam. Then with a fissure bur, section through the crown or root of each tooth four to five millimeters or more above the gingiva (if for a short coping).
2. If the canal is very narrow, drill a hole into the occlusal portion of the canal with a number one round bur approximately four millimeter deep. This will receive the metal pin.
3. Insert a flat-headed platinum-iridium pin into each canal (these pins are customarily used for pin-retained restorations). The flat head should rest on the cut surface of the root (Fig. 5-3c).
4. Tape the millimeter grid to the front of a periapical radiograph.
5. Take a radiograph of all roots with their metal pins in place.
6. Measure in millimeters the radiographic length of the root from the root apex to the bottom of the flat head (cut root surface) (Fig. 5-4).

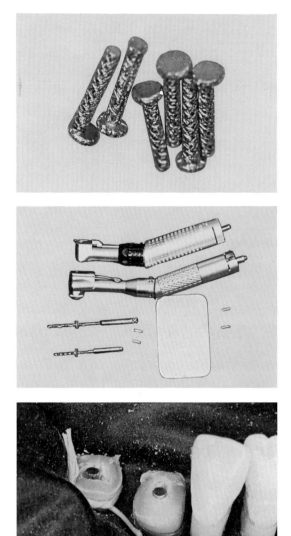

Fig. 5-3a Platinum-iridium pins used for parallel pin techniques are used as a radiographic target.

Fig. 5-3b A rectangular millimeter X-ray grid. This grid is taped to the back of a periapical radiograph prior to taking a radiograph of the root.

Fig. 5-3c A flat-headed platinum-iridium pin (used with parallel pin techniques) was inserted into each canal. The flat pin head rests on the cut surface of each root. When the canal is extremely small, drill a hole with a number one bur to receive the shaft of the pin. This pin will be used as a radiographic target for root length determination.

7. Place a rubber marker on each instrument to the proper length, less ½ mm short of the apex.
8. Instrument each canal first with a reamer, then with a file. Use the measurements obtained with the millimeter grid and metal pin, following standard endodontic procedures and progression of sizes (Fig. 5-5).

9. Frequently irrigate with 5.25% hypochlorite solution.
10. Instrument until the canal is enlarged to the desired diameter.

Mechanical Instrumentation

Instruments available for the instrumentation of the root canal should be selected

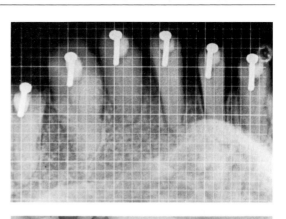

Fig. 5-4 A pin-grid radiograph records the approximate length of the cut roots. The root length is measured in millimeters by counting the millimeter spaces from the apex to the bottom surface of the flat pin head (the cut surface of the root). These measurements are used for instrumentation.

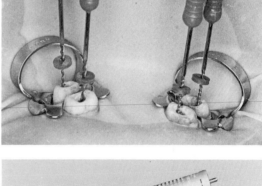

Fig. 5-5 Root canals instrumented with reamers followed by files fitted with stops for accurate instrumentation. The stops are placed on each instrument one-half millimeter short of the recorded measurements obtained with the pin-grid radiograph. In this manner there is less danger of forcing instruments beyond the root apex and simplifies obturation.

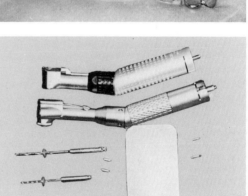

Fig. 5-6 Instruments for mechanical instrumentation of the root canal: Shown from top to bottom; giromatic contra-angle, latch-type reamer and files to be used with the giromatic contra-angle, 10:1 reduction gear contra-angle, drills used with the 10:1 reduction gear contra-angle. Also shown are the pins and millimeter grid.

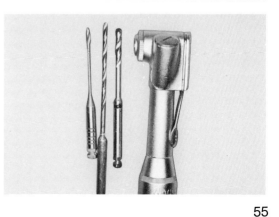

Fig. 5-7 Instruments used for direct automatic instrumentation: from right to left; 10:1 reduction gear contra-angle, para-post drill, endodontic stabilizer drill and Peso reamers.

for their effectiveness and efficiency. In addition to the customary broaches, files and reamers, the operator has available other means for instrumentation. A special giromatic contra-angle[1] that rotates in quarter rotation that can be used with latch-type endodontic reamers and files (Fig. 5-6).

The reamers, and then the file, should be carefully inserted and withdrawn as the canal is instrumented with the power-driven contra-angle. It is important to remember that the instrument sizes should be progressively changed similar to routine endodontic procedures. To do otherwise would result in a broken instrument within the canal. The disadvantage of this technique is the need for continually replacing the instruments in the contra-angle. However, this technique is applicable for use on curved roots.

The following technique is much preferred, by the authors, especially when straight or only slightly curved roots are present. A special 10:1 reduction gear contra-angle[2] is used with either endodontic stabilizer drills[3], gates glidden drills[3], peso drills[3] or para-post drills[4] (Fig. 5-7). When using this technique, select the proper sized gates glidden drill with a rubber stopper placed for accurate instrumentation. Using the stopper as a gauge, carefully drill directly into the root canal to approximately 0.5-1 mm from the root apex (Fig. 5-8). Staying short of the apex simplifies obturation and eliminates the possibility of forcing material through the apical foramen. This drill should follow the canal without perforation of the root. As you instrument the canal, drill slowly, withdrawing the drill frequently to clear the canal and drill of debris. This will prevent binding and possible drill breakage. This same technique can be followed using the endodontic stabilizer or para-post drills. In this case, first select a smaller diameter para-post drill and instru-

ment the canal to 0.5-1 mm of the apex. Then re-instrument the canal using the preferred drill to provide a larger canal to receive the guttapercha points (Fig. 5-9).

This mechanical instrumentation technique eliminates the need for constant instrument change as in the case of the giromatic-reamer-file system. This technique, however, has its limitations with very curved roots. However, where roots are only slightly curved, the drill technique will widen the curved canal and change it to a straight canal.

Use discretion in selecting the correct size drill. If the drill is too large, you may perforate the root wall.

Root Canal Irrigation and Medication

As the root canal is instrumented, frequently irrigate with 5.25% sodium hypochlorite until the root canal is enlarged to the correct size. This irrigation technique is important for removal of hard tissue debris, soft tissue remnants and necrotic materials, as well as to destroy and wash out bacteria. The canal should be dried with an absorbent point then a mild medicament such as cresatin can be used similar to conventional endodontics.

Root Canal Obturation

The instrumented root canal chamber can be filled with guttapercha, silver cones, or the endodontic material of your choice. Guttapercha is the authors' obturation material of choice. It provides a fast, efficient seal. If instrumentation is completed short of the root apex, there is virtually no danger of forcing the cone through the apex. When filling the canal with guttapercha cones, use routine endodontic techniques.

Silver cones may be preferable if abutment post hole preparations are made during the same appointment. If the coping is to be retained by a dowel, the cone should be cemented only at the apical end of the canal.

[1] Medidenta, Woodside, N.Y.
[2] Whaledent International, New York, N.Y.
[3] Medidenta, Woodside, N.Y.
[4] Whaledent International, New York, N.Y.

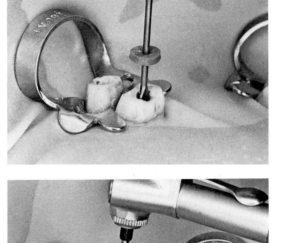

Fig. 5-8 Initial instrumentation with a small diameter Peso reamer. Preliminary instrumentation with this drill will reduce the chance of root perforation. As the canal is instrumented, the drill is repeatedly removed and cleaned to prevent it from clogging with debris. Stop instrumentation one-half to one millimeter short of the apex.

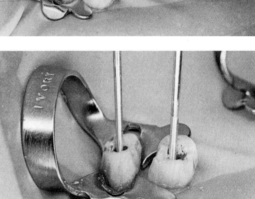

Fig. 5-9 Root canal being instrumented with a 10:1 reduction gear contra-angle and a Para-Post drill. The drill size should be no larger than the size of the obturation material to be used. A small diameter drill is used first, then followed by the desired diameter drill.

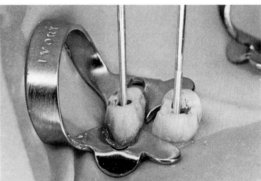

Fig. 5-10 Silver points are fitted into each root canal until a firm resistive fit is obtained.

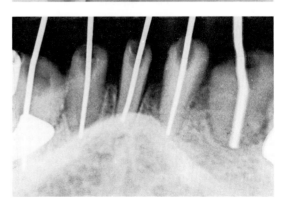

Fig. 5-11 Radiograph of roots fitted with the silver points. Notice that most canals were accurately instrumented to just near the apex. The one canal instrumented short was further adjusted.

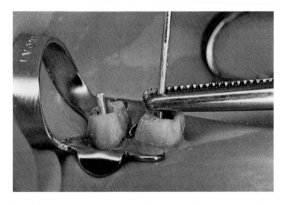

Fig. 5-12 The silver cone is clamped with a hemostat one-half millimeter above the root surface. (This allows for loss of cone length due to sectioning with a disc since part of the cone will be used as a plunger when cementing the apical portion of the cone).

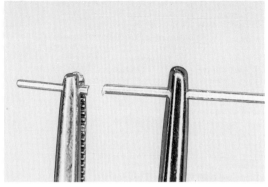

Fig. 5-13 The silver cone is sectioned with a slim disc. The end section should be long enough to seal the root end, but not too long to interfere with any dowel post preparations.

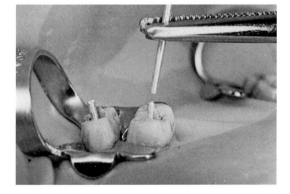

Fig. 5-14 Cement is introduced into the canal and the short cement-covered cone tip is introduced into the root canal. The larger cone section, still clamped in its original position, is used as a "measured" plunger to force the cone tip into its original position. Treated in this manner, there is little danger of forcing the cone beyond the apex, particularly if instrumentation was terminated one-half millimeter short of the apex.

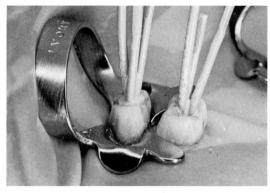

Fig. 5-15 Obturation with guttapercha cones develops an excellent apical seal. Dowel preparation should be performed later. If dowel preparations are to be performed immediately, only the apical portion should be filled with the guttapercha cone.

Here is a simple procedure for length control of silver cones:

1. Fit a silver point into each root until it fits snugly in the canal (Fig. 5-10).
2. Radiograph each root and make any adjustments necessary (Fig. 5-11). (This is only the second radiograph taken of the particular root).
3. With a hemostat, clip the silver cone ½ mm above the cut root surface (Fig. 5-12).
4. Remove the silver cone with the hemostat.
5. With another hemostat, clip the silver cone slightly above the tip of the cone.
6. Use a slim disc to section through the cone just above the second hemostat, leaving the portion to be inserted in the canal still clipped in the second hemostat (Fig. 5-13).
7. Set aside both hemostats with the silver cone sections.
8. Do the same for each root.
9. With a root canal instrument, introduce root canal sealer into each root to the correct depth.
10. Now insert the cement-covered cone tip into its respective root.
11. Use the larger portion of the sectioned cone as a measured plunger to force the small section tight into the apex (Fig. 5-14).
12. If the canal has been instrumented beyond the apex, this procedure will not force the silver cone through the apex.
13. Guttapercha cones are the material of choice for obturation when dowel preparations are drilled later (Fig. 5-15).

Chapter 6

Periodontics and the Overdenture

The object of this text is not to teach periodontics, but simply stress the importance of periodontal health for the long-term success, comfort and function of an overdenture prosthesis. Overdenture therapy lends itself to periodontal treatment and management by the general dentist. However, he should prepare himself by reading excellent texts on the subject matter and by taking appropriate courses that will prepare the practitioner in correct periodontal techniques. The general dentist, however, must have a close working relationship with the specialist for those conditions requiring special treatment.

Periodontal Consideration

Most patients who are candidates for overdenture therapy have a very debilitated oral condition, which is characterized by many missing teeth; a shifting, dropping, and extrusion of some teeth; extreme periodontal disease; and often the teeth are literally covered with calculus (Fig. 6-1). The remaining teeth have very extensive bone loss and a very unfavorable crown-root ratio. This bone picture may vary from tooth to tooth. There may be a fair to minimum bone support around some teeth, while others are just held in with skin, completely surrounded by diseased tissue.

Often those teeth with a questionable prognosis are restored with routine restorative procedures such as crown and bridge; precision partial prosthesis or some form of peridontal prosthesis. Without a proper diagnosis, this type of treatment can be a failure in a short time! Therefore, a thorough examination and accurate diagnosis are imperative.

The most important tool for such an examination is the periodontal probe (Fig. 6-2). With the periodontal probe, the dentist is able to obtain a more accurate picture of the bone and soft tissue deformities. Such an examination is made more reliable with the utilization of radiographs, tooth mobility evaluation, clinical observation of tissue color and texture, and the presence of bleeding and pus. Such a visual and clinical examination, with radiographs, study casts and periodontal probe, is used collectively to make an accurate diagnosis to formulate the most ideal treatment plan for periodontal management of the patient. Inasmuch as many of these patients have multiple dental problems to be treated, successful completion of these various treatment procedures requires a through cooperation among the patient, general dentist, periodontist, as well as the other specialists. Periodontal treatment and patient management are among the most important phases of overall overdenture treatment.

But just when is periodontal therapy completed? Often it is difficult to determine exactly when periodontal therapy should be performed for the comfort and convenience of the patient, as well as for optimum results. Each situation varies. Timing of periodontal treatment is one of the key factors for a smooth, well-coordinated treatment plan.

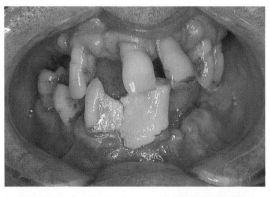

Fig. 6-1 An extreme condition of oral neglect but with teeth still not entirely hopeless for use with an overdenture. Many teeth are missing and others need to be removed due to inadequate bone support. Even though some teeth are entirely covered with calculus, they still may have adequate bone support for overdenture-supporting abutments.

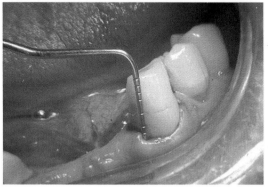

Fig. 6-2 A periodontal probe being used to thoroughly examine the extent and configuration of bone loss. A radiographic examination is incomplete without the use of such a probe.

Unfortunately, too often this therapy is performed for the convenience of the operator, rather than for the convenience and comfort of the patient.

This treatment plan may vary depending on the types of procedures required; the number of salvageable teeth; the condition and architecture of the supporting bone structure; the soft tissue character; the location of the abutments to be retained in relation to the hopeless teeth which are to be extracted; the periodontal involvement of the hopeless teeth; and whether these extractions will be accomplished prior to, during, or after periodontal therapy. Also, it should include an interim overdenture or some other form of prosthesis to be worn by the patient, if necessary.

Periodontal therapy may be performed: a) prior to any operative procedures; b) during the initial operative appoint-

ment after the hopeless teeth are removed; or c) sometime after the extractions. We will consider each of these situations separately.

Periodontal Therapy Prior to the Operative Appointments

Let us consider the situation where periodontal therapy will be performed prior to any operative procedures. When possible, this is always the best approach. Ideally, periodontal therapy should be completed 2-3 months prior to the operative appointments, such as abutment preparations. When teeth are extracted in conjunction with periodontal surgery, the soft tissue and bone of the edentulous ridge areas take much longer to heal and mature. Often it may be advisable to wait for 6 to 8 months.

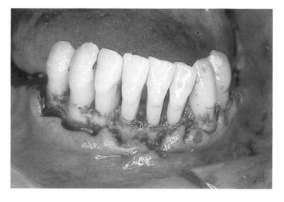

Fig. 6-3 Anterior teeth were treated periodontally after prior removal of the hopeless posterior teeth. When treated in this manner, abutment preparations are made only after complete healing and maturation of the gingival tissues. Now the patient needs to wear an interim overdenture for a minimum time and only after the anterior teeth are reduced and prepared for copings.

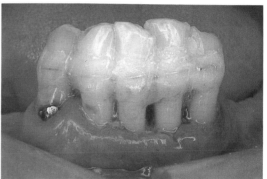

Fig. 6-4 Five lower teeth with advanced periodontal disease. This patient has never worn a lower prosthesis. The left and right cuspids and right lateral are to be retained as abutments. All of the teeth were stabilized with ligature wire covered with tooth-colored auto-polymerizing resin.

Let us consider an actual situation in which the lower arch had a full complement of teeth to be treated for overdenture therapy. All posterior teeth have a hopeless prognosis, with little or no bone support, and must be removed. The six anterior teeth are to be retained for abutments to support the overdenture.

This patient is treated much as you would treat an immediate complete-denture patient, where posterior teeth are removed first. Now, however, periodontal therapy is performed around the anterior teeth (Fig. 6-3).

The patient needs no interim overdenture during the healing stage, since the patient has the six anterior teeth for function and cosmetics. Now an interim overdenture is necessary only after the abutment teeth are prepared for the overdenture. Treating the teeth periodontally in this manner permits the interim overdenture to be worn for a much shorter time, only during the final phase of treatment after the teeth have been reduced.

Periodontal therapy should also be performed initially wherever you have retained vital abutments and no interim prosthesis is necessary for appearance, for example: when the abutments will remain vital, requiring long copings; or where a removable prosthesis is already being used or can be fabricated to fit around the periodontally treated teeth until healing and maturation.

Consider another situation where there are lower anterior teeth present (Fig. 6-4).

The centrals and left lateral have no bone support and the roots are completely surrounded by diseased tissue. The cuspids and right lateral will be retained and the others removed. To effectively treat the abutment teeth, the other teeth must be removed first. This particular patient was not wearing a prosthesis for posterior replacement, so there is no reason to provide one after periodontal treatment during the healing period. This case was treated periodontally in this manner: To facilitate periodontal therapy and to eliminate the need for an interim overdenture during the healing period, the centrals and left lateral were splinted to the other teeth with wire and resin. Next, the roots of the teeth to be removed were sectioned and the root tips removed, leaving only the crowns splinted to the other teeth for esthetics. These splinted teeth were retained in this manner until all tissues healed (Fig. 6-5). This simple technique eliminated the need for the patient to wear and adjust to an interim overdenture for the two to three months necessary for healing and maturation of tissues.

Periodontal Therapy during Operative Appointments

The more complex treatment situations are those in which you are confronted with multiple dental problems, where the treatment of one depends upon the successful treatment of the other. Generally a few teeth will be retained for abutments; others will be extracted. The teeth that are to be removed may be so involved with periodontal disease that it is difficult to treat the neighboring teeth periodontally. It then becomes imperative that the hopeless teeth be removed just before periodontal surgery.

Periodontal Surgery sometime after Extractions

Sometimes improved periodontal results are obtained if these hopeless teeth are removed early – several months prior to periodontal therapy or the operative phase. This allows time for the filling-in of bone in the edentulous areas during the healing process. Periodontal therapy is then performed months later around the remaining abut-

ment teeth. But now around abutment teeth that has had some filling-in of bone. An interim removable appliance may or may not be necessary, depending on whether the abutment teeth have been reduced or have been retained intact.

Treatment of the most Common Periodontal Condition

Let us consider a situation in which the abutment teeth have minimal bone support, the teeth must be reduced to produce a favorable crown and root ratio, endodontics will be necessary, hopeless teeth will be extracted and interim prosthesis is to be inserted after periodontal surgery. The following is an outline of the procedure generally followed by the author when periodontal therapy is performed during the initial operative appointment.

1. Initially there must be extensive home care instruction after thorough prophylaxis, soft tissue curettage and root planning.
2. During the initial operative appointment the abutment teeth are reduced, or roughly prepared according to the coping types selected. If the abutments are to remain vital, they will need some form of temporary coverage to eliminate sensitivity. If they are reduced to the level of the gingiva, they must be treated endodontally. When there is minimal bone support the teeth are reduced appropriately to the gingiva. For example, the teeth are reduced about 1 to 2 millimeters (mm) above the gingival margin with a fissure bur; then the occlusal portion of the root pulp chamber is widened with a No. 4 bur to about 3 to 4 mm deep (this provides room for medicament and a temporary stopping).
3. Endodontic therapy is initiated or completed.
4. The hopeless teeth are removed.
5. The abutment teeth are rough-prepared.

Fig. 6-5 Roots of teeth to be removed were sectioned and their root tips removed, leaving their crowns splinted to the other teeth. The remaining teeth were treated periodontally. Since the patient had not worn a previous prosthesis, no interim appliance was provided during healing and tissue-maturation stage. Treated in this manner, the patient will require an interim overdenture for a very minimal time and only after the remaining teeth are prepared.

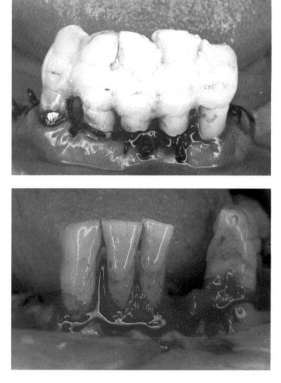

Fig. 6-6 Conservative osseous and soft-tissue surgery around the lower teeth with extreme lingual bone loss. Radical osseous contouring to entirely remove the bony defects would require removal of much of the remaining bone support, further weakening the already weak abutment.

6. Periodontal surgery is completed around the retained abutments.
7. Finally, an interim overdenture is inserted both as a bandage and to provide the function, comfort and esthetic requirements of the patient.

Periodontal Therapy

No restorative dentistry should be performed on periodontally diseased abutment teeth. Therefore, all periodontal problems should be eliminated to improve the long-range prognosis of these "questionable" teeth. The periodontal therapy techniques should conserve as much bone support and attached gingiva as is possible. Although periodontal therapy should always consist of sound principles, some variation in standard technique seems to be indicated (from that normally performed on teeth with much bone support) for the highly unstable teeth generally encountered in overdenture prosthodontics. Since there is only minimal bone support remaining, the dentist cannot afford to destroy additional alveolar root support with radical bone – contouring techniques. It is, therefore, ill-advised to contour excessively osseous defects simply to make a more favorable bony contour. To do so would require the removal of much of the root supporting bone that remains. With this in mind, conservation in soft tissue and osseous surgery is of utmost importance (Fig. 6-6).

Since such bone conservation is imperative, periodontal surgery will leave less than ideal osseous and soft tissue contour around the abutment teeth. This can readily be compensated by specially contoured copings designed for ideal periodontal health and

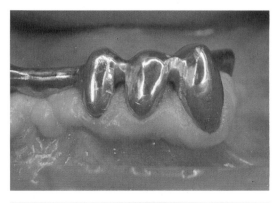

Fig. 6-7 Copings contoured into the periodontal defects to compensate for extensive tissue destruction here. This helps to prevent additional tissue destruction. Copings are tapering, not over-contoured, and shaped into the defects both facially and lingually. Note the high interproximal contours that follow the gingival outline. The interproximal embrasures are designed for periodontal health.

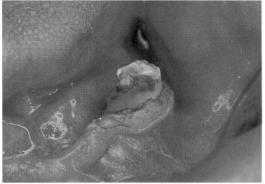

Fig. 6-8 Soft tissue defects removed from around the lower cuspid by a simple gingivectomy. When this excess of soft tissue is not involved with bony defects, it can be removed with a sharp periodontal knife or even electrosurgically.

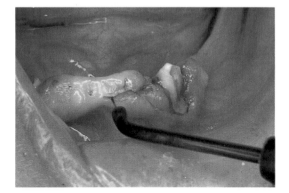

Fig. 6-9 Electrosurgery being used to remove loose superfluous tissue covering the lower anterior alveolar ridge. This will improve the soft-tissue support for the overdenture.

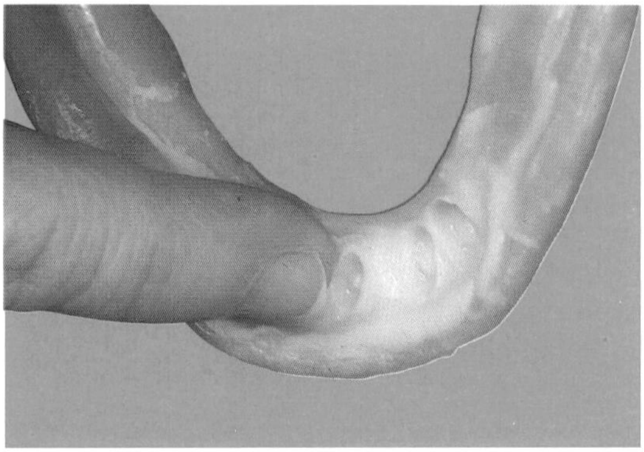

Fig. 6-10 Readapting the thin flashes of soft liner back into the denture. These flashes were produced when the interim overdenture was fitted with the soft liner over the periodontal surgical site. If the soft liner is left in this manner, very poor periodontal results can be expected. Therefore it must be readapted with the fingers. The interim overdenture is inserted and removed several times while continually readapting the soft relining material. This molds the tissue conditioning material around the surgical site apically positioning the soft tissue around the abutments.

maintenance. Here you see a few examples. Notice the crowns have been contoured to compensate for this less-than-desirable bone and soft tissue contour and anatomy (Fig. 6-7).

When there is inadequate attached gingiva, grafts should be utilized whenever possible to improve the attached gingival zone. Where only a few teeth remain and there are no significant osseous deformities, soft tissue defects can frequently be corrected by simple gingivectomy techniques using either periodontal cutting instruments or with electrosurgery (Fig. 6-8). Superfluous tissue covering the alveolar ridge should also be removed to improve the overdenture foundation. Such tissue is readily removed with electrosurgery (Fig. 6-9).

Periodontal Surgery Management with Interim Overdentures

A transitional overdenture is the most valuable tool to treat the overdenture patient in an efficient, controlled, expeditious manner. This transitional overdenture, as a management vehicle, transforms the many complicated procedures into more manageable tasks. It is also a valuable tool used to coordinate treatment with the various specialists such as the oral surgeon, periodontist, and the endodontist. When there are teeth to be retained, numerous teeth that are to be extracted; and when it would be difficult to treat them periodontally without the prior removal of the hopeless teeth – the transitional overdenture comes into play.

Now let us consider the proper use of the interim or transitional overdenture. The dentist should have available a previously constructed interim overdenture fabricated before the initial operative appointment. The construction of this overdenture will be discussed in more detail in a later chapter.

Acrylic teeth should be positioned over each abutment. After tooth reduction, endodontics, extractions, and periodontal therapy, partially hollow out the base of the denture and resin denture teeth over the abutments, and insert the overdenture. If it does not sit passively, but rather impinges on the abutments, the denture teeth must be hollowed even more.

The interim overdenture is both prosthesis and periodontal dressing. The success of the periodontal therapy depends to a great degree on how well you adjust the interim overdenture to the surgical site. This is accomplished in this manner:

1. After the general fit has been adjusted by properly hollowing the area over each abutment, place a mix of soft reline material[1] inside the denture.
2. Insert the overdenture and have the patient close gently into occlusion.
3. Immediately remove the overdenture and eliminate excessive flash material over the ridge area of the prosthesis.
4. Examine the overdenture for extruding flashes of material between the surgical flaps and around the abutments. This flash must be eliminated or it will prevent proper tissue healing and tissue adaptation. Using a wet finger, push all such flash back into the overdenture (Fig. 6-10).
5. Reinsert the overdenture and again have the patient close into occlusion. This will adapt the soft reline material around the abutments apically, positioning the surgical flaps for ideal gingival form.
6. Remove the overdenture and repeat steps 4 and 5.

After the patient has worn this appliance for a long time, the soft relining material soon becomes hard and irritating to the tissues. Bacteria will soon be incorporated into the porous materials. This is not conducive to

[1] Coe Comfort, Coe Laboratories, Inc., Chicago, Ill.

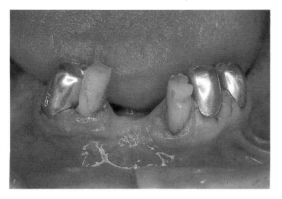

Fig. 6-11a Trimmed, shaped and contoured aluminum crowns fitted to vital teeth prepared for long copings. The copings are cemented with a medicinal cement to prevent sensitivity.

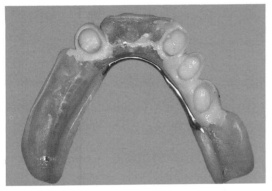

Fig. 6-11b These temporary crowns act as copings to support the interim overdenture adapted over them with auto-polymerizing resin.

good healing processes. If the patient is to wear this denture for a long time, the old relining material should be replaced with new material. Change this material weekly for the first two weeks then in two weeks, then monthly.

Interim Overdentures, Vital Abutments and Periodontal Management

A special transitional overdenture management problem exists when the abutments are prepared as vital abutments for long copings. If abutments are left uncovered, there will be a sensitivity problem. Of course, for the management of the individual abutments, they must be provided with some form of temporary coverage to prevent this pulpal sensitivity.

One method of treatment is to fit these abutments with temporary acrylic crowns. Then an interim prosthesis is fitted around these temporary crowns. This, however, is more time-consuming and is associated with adjustment problems.

A better treatment for such a situation is to cover these teeth with aluminum crowns. These should be carefully adapted, tapered, and the margins smoothed to act as temporary copings (Fig. 6-11a). Then the transitional overdenture is adapted and relined to fit over these covered teeth (Fig. 6-11b). This serves several purposes – the cemented temporary coverage prevents abutment sensitivity; the interim overdenture again acts as a periodontal dressing; and the tapered aluminum crowns act as supporting and retaining copings.

Chapter 7

Interim or Transitional Overdentures

Management Techniques

As discussed earlier, an interim or transitional overdenture is one of the most important and useful devices for efficient management of overdenture techniques. These procedures require time, organization, and the need to manage these various steps for the comfort and convenience of the patient and the dentist. Without the use of an interim overdenture, these treatment procedures would be difficult to manage. The dentist would soon be discouraged from providing overdenture service for his patients.

Functions of Interim Overdentures

An interim or transitional overdenture serves many functions:

1. Makes possible the removal of hopeless teeth for the comfort, function and appearance of the patient during treatment.
2. Acts as a bandage after periodontal surgery.
3. Provides an opportunity for a team approach when referring these patients to the various specialists.
4. Endodontics is simplified by elimination of the clinical crown, providing for more direct access and ease of instrumentation during root canal therapy.
5. It is the device used so that endodontics can be completed more leisurely and

through roots by the specialist or general dentist.
6. The retained abutment tooth or roots can be more readily evaluated for their long-term prognosis after periodontal therapy and subsequent healing.
7. The final preparation of the abutment teeth can be made while the interim overdenture is still being worn.
8. The primary copings, and/or attachments, can be cemented and customized to fit the interim overdenture. Now a master impression can be taken to form a cast for fabrication of the overlay prosthesis.
9. Maintains interocclusal relationship during treatment.
10. Acts as a transitional prosthesis for patient acceptance.
11. Helps to stabilize and support the weak abutments after surgery.

A variety of techniques are available for fabricating interim overdentures: modification of an existing prosthesis, autopolymer resin overdentures, or heat-cured resin techniques.

Modification of Existing Prosthesis

The simplest procedure is to modify an existing removable prosthesis as an interim overdenture (Fig. 7-1a). This is always recommended, for it reduces the patient's cost. It also utilizes a prosthesis that the

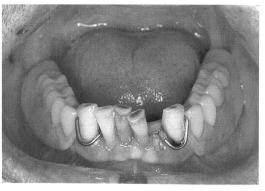

Fig. 7-1a An existing partial denture can be modified to serve as an interim overdenture.

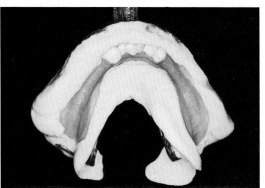

Fig. 7-1b Tooth-colored auto-polymerizing resin placed into the impression void representing the natural dentition.

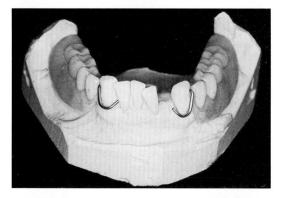

Fig. 7-1c After the resin hardened, stone was poured into the remainder of the impression, to produce a stone cast with tooth-colored resin teeth. The partial removed with the impression becomes a part of the cast.

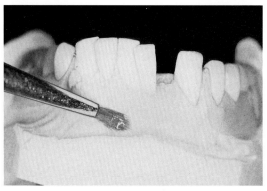

Fig. 7-1d The exposed stone is coated with a separating medium.

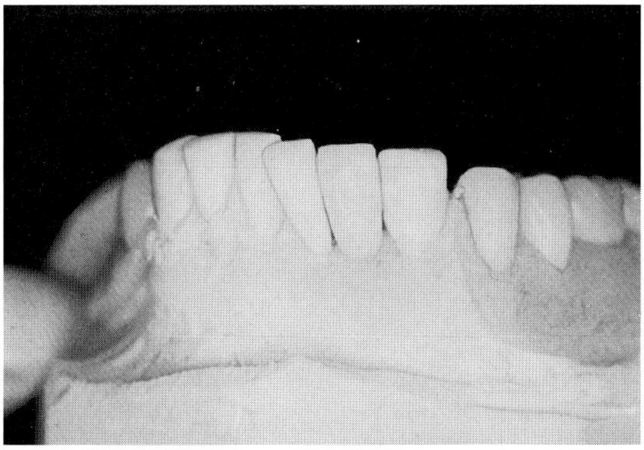

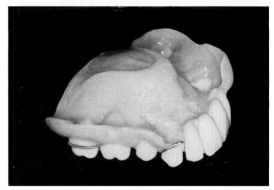

Fig. 7-1e   Missing teeth replaced with resin denture teeth.

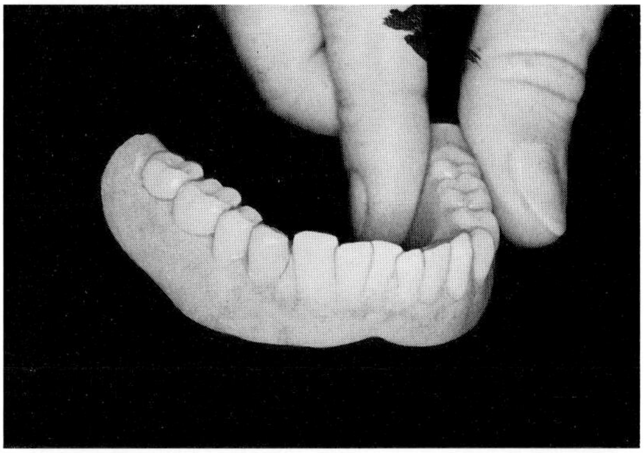

Fig. 7-1f   Tissue-colored auto-polymerizing resin was added to build a flange to the original prosthesis, transforming the original prosthesis into an interim overdenture.

Fig. 7-1g   A completed interim overdenture ready for insertion. The area over each abutment tooth is hollowed out to fit over the semi-prepared abutments. The prosthesis should be fitted in the mouth and checked for occlusion and non-impingement over the abutments.

patient has been accustomed to and familiar with. This is a procedure easily performed, in the office, by the dental auxiliary. It may even be fabricated during the initial operative appointment.

Used with Non-Vital Abutments

1. With the removable partial denture in place and the clasp loosened, take an alginate impression of the remaining teeth, the partial and the dental arch.
2. Remove the set impression with the removable partial embeded.
3. Place tooth-colored auto-polymer resin mix such as jet[1] into the voids produced by the natural dentition (Fig. 7-1b).
4. Place the impression in a humidor or pressure flask until the resin cures.
5. Fill the remaining impression and partial denture with model stone. This forms a cast with the partial in place and the natural teeth in plastic (Fig. 7-1c).
6. Break off all exposed clasps.
7. Paint the exposed set stone with a separating media in the denture flange area to be built (Fig. 7-1d).
8. Replace any missing teeth with an appropriate acrylic denture tooth. These can be temporarily held in place by securing the teeth with a small amount of sticky wax added to the occlusal edges (Fig. 7-1e).
9. Moisten a brush with liquid monimer, pick up a drop of perm[2] powder and deposit the moist mass on the flangeless area of the cast. Continue adding sufficient resin up and around the neck of each resin tooth and any added denture teeth (Fig. 7-1f).
10. Before the resin is completely polymerized, place the cast in a pressure tank under 30 pounds of pressure until completely polymerized.

11. Remove the interim overdenture modification from the cast, adjust the flange, festoon around the necks of the added teeth, and polish.
12. Hollow out each resin tooth sufficiently to fit over the abutment teeth. The interim overdenture is now ready for use after extraction of all hopeless teeth and after periodontal surgery (Fig. 7-1g).

Used with Vital Abutments

1. Take an accurate alginate impression of the dental arch with the partial denture in place.
2. Remove the set impression with the partial retained in the impression and place in a humidor.
3. Prepare the abutments for long copings.
4. Select the correct size aluminum shell crown, trim, adapt to the gingival margin, and cement on the abutment tooth with a medicated cement. These covered abutments will act as copings to support the interim overdenture (Fig. 7-2).
5. Extract the hopeless teeth and perform periodontal surgery.
6. Place tooth-colored acrylic resin in the voids produced by the abutment teeth.
7. After soft polymerization of the resin material, place the impression with the retained partial in the mouth over the edentulous areas and abutment preparations.
8. Remove, and reinsert the impression continuously until the resin sets. The tooth-colored resin forms secondary copings over the aluminum primary copings.
9. After the resin hardens, remove the modified partial from the impression and shape the resin teeth as you would any temporary resin crowns, and polish. The interim overdenture is ready for use (Fig. 7-3).

Note! A flange is seldom used with this technique, but if necessary it may be added as in the previous procedure.

[1] Lang. Dental Mfg., Co., Chicago, Ill.
[2] Hygienic Dental Mfg., Co., Akron, Ohio

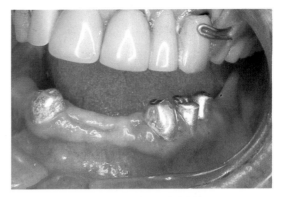

Fig. 7-2 An existing prosthesis modified with tooth-colored auto-polymerizing resin to fit over aluminum crown copings.

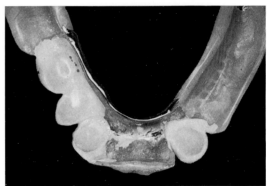

Fig. 7-3 An existing removable partial denture modified with tooth-colored resin to fit over aluminum crowns. The resin secondary coping fits over the aluminum crown as do temporary resin crowns.

Immediate Interim Overdenture Using Denture Teeth

A conventional interim overdenture can be fabricated much as you would a complete denture.

Heat-Cured Packing Technique

1. Take an impression of both arches for casts with alginate or reversible hydro-colloid material. The models are articulated on an appropriate articulator with accurate occlussal records and used for study casts and fabrication of interim overdentures.
2. Remove the teeth to be extracted from the cast.
3. Roughly prepare the abutment teeth on the cast to approximately the preparation to be made in the mouth later (Fig. 7-4).

4. Grind out acrylic denture teeth to fit over the rough stone preparation and set in occlusion.
5. Replace the teeth to be extracted with denture teeth.
6. Wax up and festoon the denture flanges (Fig. 7-5).
7. Flask, pack, cure and finish the case.

Auto-Polymerizing Technique

Interim overdentures may also be fabricated using some type of auto-polymerizing pour procedure, such as Pronto[1], Coe[2] or the Densply's Tru-Pour technique[3].
The latter technique (Densply's Tru-Pour) is used by the authors and is a technique easily mastered by the dental auxiliary. A thorough

[1] Vernon – Benstoff Co., Inc., Albany, N.Y.
[2] Coe Laboratories, Chicago, Ill.
[3] Densply International Inc., York, Pa.

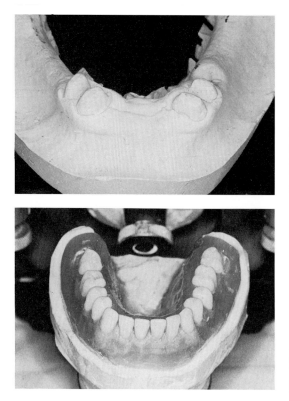

Fig. 7-4   Cast for fabrication of an interim over-denture. The teeth to be extracted are removed from the cast. The prepared abutment teeth on the cast are reduced and rough-prepared similar to that in the mouth.

Fig. 7-5   The interim overdenture with the denture teeth set up, waxed, festooned and ready for processing.

step-by-step procedure may be obtained from the manufacturer.

Other Interim Overdenture Considerations

Additional modifications in interim overdenture use and technique is limited only by one's own imagination and ingenuity. In fact, interim overdentures may eventually become the final prosthesis. Or, it may even be modified to act as a complete denture. In this later case, the interim overdenture should be fabricated without a metal framework and processed with a more durable resin material rather than with auto-polymerizing resin.

To transform this interim prosthesis into an attachment-retained prosthesis, the prosthesis can be fitted over the copings with self-curing resin. The clip, or female, portion of any attachment now may be processed into the tissue side of the prosthesis directly in the mouth.

The interim prosthesis may also be modified to function as a "spare" overdenture by routine clinical and laboratory procedures.

Chapter 8

Abutment Preparations and Coping Consideration

Abutment preparations are critical for esthetics, coping retention, and a favorable crown-root ratio. Final abutment preparations are made only after healing and maturation of tissues, after surgery. Wait at least 2 to 3 months for periodontal healing and maturation of tissues. Wait 6 to 8 months if numerous extractions were involved. You will notice that now the abutments extend further above the gingiva than when first reduced. They will need to be reduced farther now. The abutment design starts with an accurate examination, diagnosis, and treatment plan. You must have a mental image of this preparation before even the initial reduction. It will depend upon the coping type to be constructed. Coping types, and preparations, will be determined by the following factors:

- Number of abutments used.
- Amount of bone support.
- The need for more favorable crown-root ratio.
- Opposing dentition (natural dentition, another overdenture, a complete denture, etc.).
- Vertical space available.
- Will there be copings?
- Will there be attachments?
- What kind of attachments?

Coping types and abutment preparations depend on many of these factors. These preparations can often determine the success or failure of the overdenture treatment. Each of the four types of primary copings requires a special preparation.

Short Preparations (non-vital)

1. For bare root abutments.
2. For short copings.

Medium-Short Preparations (non-vital)

1. For bare root abutments.
2. For medium-short copings.

Medium Preparation (vital or non-vital)

1. For medium size copings.

Long Preparations (vital)

1. Long copings with resin secondary copings.
2. Long copings with attachments.
3. Long copings to be used with metal secondary copings.

The preparations summarized above, and copings associated with each, will be discussed in more detail. The short preparation is the one most commonly used in overdenture therapy. As we have already discussed, the typical abutment suffers extreme bone loss, so the crown must be reduced close to the gingiva to create a favorable crown-root ratio. There are two types of short abutments:

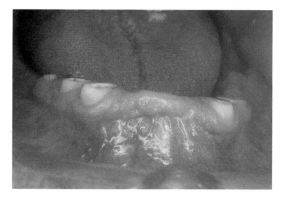

Fig. 8-1a Teeth reduced close to the gingiva and used as bare-root abutments to support an overdenture.

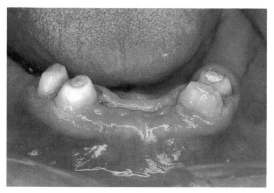

Fig. 8-1b Bare-root abutments four to five millimeters long with slightly parallel proximal walls designed for retention.

Short Preparation for Bare-Root Abutment

Such an abutment conserves the alveolar ridge, as well as provide support, but it does not provide retention.

The occlusal contour should be slightly convex with the occlusal surface following the contour of the alveolar ridge. Some operators prepare a slight concavity into the root surface to provide additional room for set up of the denture teeth. However, sufficient room for denture teeth is not normally a problem in such a situation. The overall occlusal height should be approximately 1-2 millimeters (mm) (Fig. 8-1a). Bare-root abutments used for retention are slightly longer (4-5 millimeters, Fig. 8-1b). The occlusal opening of the root canal should be restored with silver amalgam. Highly polish the occlusal surface of the root and silver amalgam, using in succession a fine sandpaper disc,

fine rubber point, and a rubber disc, first with pumice and finally with zinc oxide powder.

Short Preparation for Short Copings

This is the most common overdenture abutment preparation. When used without a stud or bar attachment, the abutment, fitted with a short coping, conserves the alveolar ridge and provides support. When fitted with an attachment it will also retain the overlay prosthesis (Fig. 8-2). It is prepared in this manner:

1. Prior to periodontal surgery, cut partly through the clinical crown of the tooth with a carbide fissure bur facially, lingually and 1 to 2 mm above the gingival margin (of course this tooth is treated endodontically).

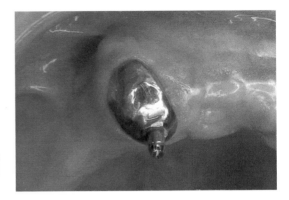

Fig. 8-2 Preparation for short copings to provide the most favorable crown-root ratio. When fitted with attachment, retention is provided.

2. After periodontal therapy, healing and maturation of tissue, the tooth is now much higher above the gingival tissues and must again be reduced (Fig. 8-3a).
3. With a carbide fissure or diamond bur, reduce and shape the occlusal surface of the root to about 1 to 2mm above the gingival margin. Use the contour of the alveolar ridge as your guide (Fig. 8-3b).
   a) On the lower ridge where the gingival margin is even and uniform, the occlusal cut should be rather uniform. This will fulfill the demands of favorable crown-root ratio and esthetics. Where the gingival margin is even facially and lingually, the root surface may be flat or slightly convex (Fig. 8-4a).
   b) On the lower ridge where there is extensive bone loss lingually, do not follow the gingiva lingually, but just round off the occlusal corner of the preparation here (Fig. 8-4b).
   c) In the upper anterior area where esthetics requirement is very critical, it is very important to follow the contour of the ridge, particularly along the facial aspect of the ridge (Fig. 8-4c). There must be adequate reduction facially to allow room for the coping as well as for the denture teeth (Fig. 8-4d).
4. The short proximal walls of the preparation should be as parallel as possible to provide maximum retention but without

undercut areas. Where copings are to be connected, proximal walls of abutments should be closely parallel.
5. There should be either a feather edge or champfer margin extending slightly below the crest of the gingiva (Fig. 8-5). Generally there is inadequate root diameter to develop a heavy shoulder preparation with a bevel.
6. Prepare a 1 mm indentation (in the form of a +) on the occlusal surface (Fig. 8-6). This provides for added thickness and strength here on the thin diaphragm of the gold coping. It also aids in the orientation of the coping on the root during cementation.
7. If you are using posts or pins for coping retention, prepare the holes. (See "Posts and Pins," chapter 9.)
8. When dowel retention is used for the coping, the occlusal of the post hole should be enlarged with a No. 6 bur to about half the diameter of the bur. A No. 4 bur may be used with a very narrow root and a No. 8 bur with a larger root. This depression adds strength to the post (Fig. 8-7).
9. Lastly, smooth all surfaces with a fine grit diamond bur.

Medium-Short Preparation with Non-Vital Teeth

Medium-short preparations may be left bare or restored with cast copings.

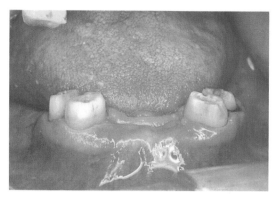

Fig. 8-3a   The abutment teeth were reduced to the level of the gingiva before periodontal surgery. Note that they now extend substantially higher after healing and maturation of the gingival tissues. These abutments must now be reduced further.

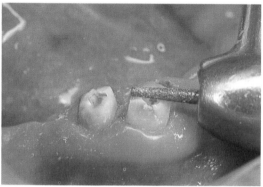

Fig. 8-3b   A diamond bur being used to reduce the abutments to one to two millimeters above the gingiva. This extreme reduction is necessary to improve the crown-root ratio.

Medium-Short Preparations for Bare-Root Abutments

Such a preparation is indicated when there is sufficient bone support and when copings are not made for economical reasons. Bare roots provide support and some retention. The overall form is bullet-like or conical. The gingival half of the root may have slightly parallel walls for minimum retention (Fig. 8-8). It can taper to a cone form in the occlusal half. Actually, the completed preparation would be similar to a cast coping designed for retention. The canal opening is then filled with silver and all surfaces are highly polished.

Medium-Short Preparations for Copings

Medium-short preparations can be used with copings when more favorable crown-root ratio is still desirable, but a slightly higher preparation is made to improve the retention of the coping on the abutment. Such a preparation is indicated when the medium-short coping is to be used with bar attachments, or when such splinted multiple copings require favorable embrasures for periodontal health (Fig. 8-9). Follow these steps for making the medium-short preparations for copings:

1. After periodontal healing, reduce the occlusal surface to approximately 3 to 4 mm above the gingival margin.
2. The facial and lingual preparations (particularly the facial surface) are made more tapered. This facial reduction provides room for an esthetic set-up of the denture teeth. The gingival half of the proximal walls is prepared more parallel but tapering occlusally in the occlusal half. The marginal preparation extends

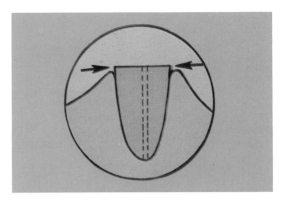

Fig. 8-4a   The occlusal surface closely follows the alveolar ridge contour. When the gingiva crest is uniform in height, the abutment surface is slightly convex or even flat.

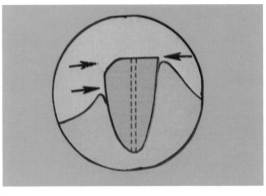

Fig. 8-4b   When extensive bone loss is present lingually, just round off the occlusal lingual corner, as shown in this illustration.

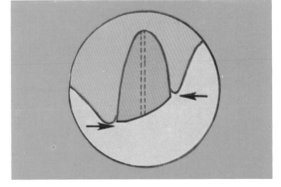

Fig. 8-4c   An illustration of a recommended maxillary anterior short preparation. It must follow the entire facial contour for maximum room for the anterior teeth.

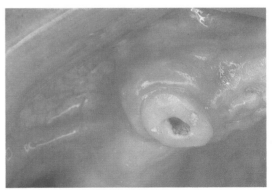

Fig. 8-4d   A typical example of the degree of reduction for upper anterior abutments.

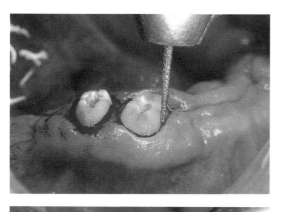

Fig. 8-5 Proximal preparation being made with a fine-grit diamond bur. The short proximal walls should be closely parallel to maximize coping retention. A chamfer margin is preferred; however, for narrow roots a feathered-edge margin preparation is acceptable.

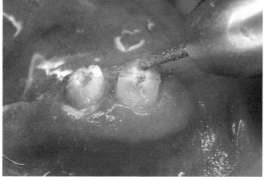

Fig. 8-6 A one millimeter indentation in the form of an "X" is prepared into the root face. An inverted cone carbide bur or the corner of a flat-ended diamond can be used. This indentation provides room for added thickness of the coping diaphragm for greater strength. It also aids in the orientation of the coping on the abutment.

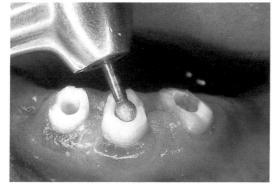

Fig. 8-7 The top of the dowel preparation is enlarged with a number six or eight bur. This additional space provides added thickness and subsequent strength to the cast dowel. If a prefabricated dowel is used, there is a more definite bond to the dowel here.

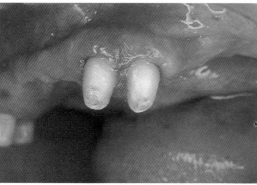

Fig. 8-8 Bare roots prepared to function as medium-short copings for improved retention of the overdenture. The occlusal opening of the root canal can be restored with silver amalgam. It is bullet-like in overall contour with the gingival half of the proximal walls slightly parallel. The occlusal portion is conical.

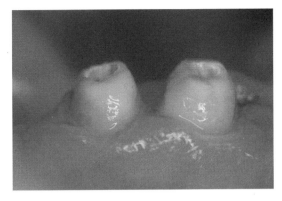

Fig. 8-9 Medium-short abutments prepared to receive medium-short copings. The root is prepared approximately four to five millimeters high with a general tapering form facially-lingually. The gingival half of the proximal walls are more parallel for better retention of the copings on the abutment.

just below the crest of the gingiva, and may be a feathered edge or a chamfer-type of margin.
3. Auxiliary retention for the coping on the abutment is still recommended for such a preparation and will be considered later.

Medium Coping Preparation for Vital or Non-Vital Teeth

Often there is adequate root support, so extreme reduction of a tooth to produce maximum favorable crown-root ratio is not necessary (the tooth is devitalized); or when the pulp has receded over the years, a medium preparation may permit you to reduce crown-root ratio somewhat without devitalizing the tooth. These preparations are similar in all respects to the procedure for medium-short preparations but are slightly longer (Fig. 8-10a). Here again, the facial and lingual surfaces are very tapering, with most reduction done at the expense of the facial surface for esthetics.

These copings may be utilized for a simple telescopic overdenture to provide retention by the proximal wall parallelism (Fig. 8-10b); or they may be used with auxiliary retention devices such as bars (Fig. 8-10c), Ipsoclips, IC attachments (Fig. 8-10d), Octalinks, Cekas, etc. Stud attachments even may be cantilevered off such copings (Fig. 8-10e). A

thorough discussion of these attachments will be included later in the text.

Long Preparations with Vital Teeth

There are two preparation designs for long copings: (1) one should be used when the acrylic denture base will sit directly over the primary coping; (2) the other should be used when a metal or porcelain-to-metal secondary coping will telescope over the primary coping.

Long Primary Coping Preparations for Use with an Acrylic Resin Secondary Coping

These preparations are made for copings with an overall tapering form (Fig. 8-11a). Its use is indicated for telescopic overdentures, retained with proximal wall parallelism, or, with auxiliary attachments such as bars, Ipsoclips, IC attachments, Octalinks, Cekas, etc. Make the preparation in this manner (Fig. 8-11b):

1. Reduce the clinical crown apically as far as possible without causing pulp exposure.
2. Develop a definite taper facially and lingually, with more reduction faciallly. This permits more room anteriorly for the

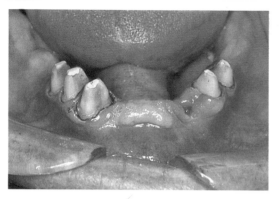

Fig. 8-10a   Abutment preparation for medium copings prepared similar to the medium-short form but slightly longer (4-6 millimeters).

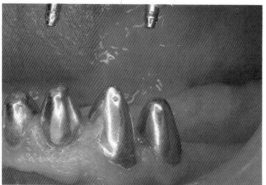

Fig. 8-10b   These medium copings provide support and retention for a telescopic overdenture.

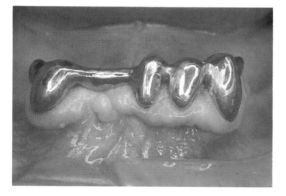

Fig. 8-10c   Medium copings splinted with a bar attachment. Retention is provided primarily by the bar. The copings are very tapered in form.

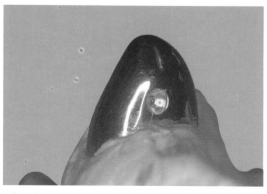

Fig. 8-10d   Medium coping with a round depression that will be engaged by the plunger of a spring-loaded attachment.

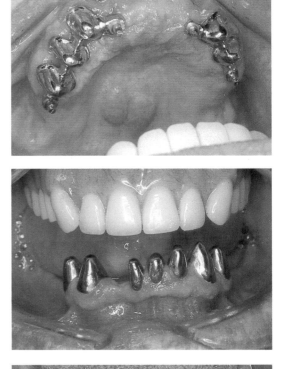

Fig. 8-10e   Studs cantilevered distal to medium copings for additional retention.

Fig. 8-11a   Long copings used to support an overdenture with a resin denture base.

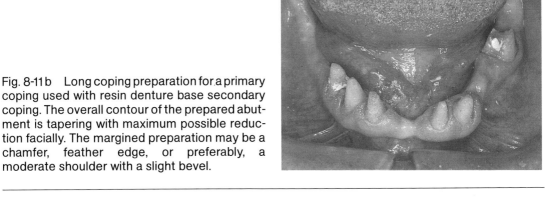

Fig. 8-11b   Long coping preparation for a primary coping used with resin denture base secondary coping. The overall contour of the prepared abutment is tapering with maximum possible reduction facially. The margined preparation may be a chamfer, feather edge, or preferably, a moderate shoulder with a slight bevel.

esthetic set-up of the denture teeth. This is often a problem with long coping telescopic overdenture.

3. The gingival halves of the proximal wall should be approximately parallel to each other. The upper ½ of the walls should taper toward the occlusal.

4. A feathered edge, chamfer, or shoulder preparation with a slight bevel may be

used. The latter margin preparation is the treatment of choice.

Preparations for Long Primary Coping to be Used with Metal Secondary Copings (Fig. 8-12a).

Such an abutment tooth is prepared to receive a long primary coping which will be

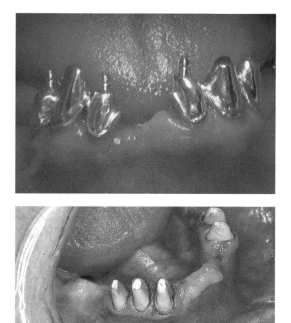

Fig. 8-12a   Shouldered long copings to fit a porcelain-to-metal secondary coping.

Fig. 8-12b   Abutments prepared to receive a shouldered primary coping and a porcelain-to-metal secondary coping. This preparation is similar to that shown in Fig. 8-11, but with a heavy shoulder. The shoulder is prepared slightly below the crest of the gingiva. Therefore the coping shoulder can be located just above the crest of the gingiva.

covered by a metal or a porcelain-to-metal secondary coping. The primary coping has a heavy shoulder that is located at the gingival crest. Since basically a double crown is to be placed over the abutment, the tooth must be reduced more extensively on all axial surfaces. A definite heavy shoulder with a beveled margin is prepared completely around the tooth (Fig. 8-12b). The proximal and lingual shoulder preparation need not be as extensive as the facial surface. Such a preparation will provide adequate room for the thickness of the primary and secondary coping. The shoulder should follow the contour of the gingival margin and is extended just below its crest.

Chapter 9

Coping Retention

Overdenture prosthetics has many similarities to basic restorative dental procedures. It therefore has similar requirements – such as the necessity for a secure fit of the casting on the abutment teeth and ability of the casting to withstand torquing actions transmitted by the removable prosthesis. Forces applied by the removable prosthesis during function – or on removal – tends to loosen the copings from the roots. Therefore it is of utmost importance that copings be provided with adequate retention to resist dislodgement.

Retention of copings on teeth prepared for long copings, or even medium copings normally is not a problem. The frictional retention of the coping with the longer axial walls of the preparation provides adequate retention. With short copings, the axial walls of the preparation may be only a few millimeters in length. The frictional retention of these limited axial walls is inadequate to retain short copings. Short copings should have additional auxiliary retention to minimize this problem with overdenture treatment. Retention can be provided with any of the following methods:

– Posts (tapered, parallel walled, stepped, threaded)
– Parallel pins
– Non-parallel pins
– Post-pin combinations
– Threaded screw systems
– Custom dowels

Dowel (Post) Retention

A variety of techniques and procedures are available for fabricating copings with dowels for added retention. Most systems utilize special sizing drills and/or reamers to prepare the canal for a sized post. The design of these posts may vary from a tapered form, to a parallel-wall form, to a stepped form, or even a threaded form.

Non-Parallel Posts

Individual dowel-retained copings not splinted together do not require parallel dowel preparations as the copings will be cemented separately. In this case, the canals can be prepared "free-hand" using any type of post system.

Parallel Posts

Where multiple abutments are to be splinted, parallelism of the posts is mandatory. Free-hand preparation of canals to receive parallel-walled dowels is often difficult. Therefore a tapered dowel is recommended for free-hand drilling of parallel canals.

Free-Hand Drilling for Parallel Tapered Post Holes

When parallel post holes are prepared free-hand, the taper of the canal compensates for some of the error of paralleling the drill "free-hand." Any of the following tapered post systems may be used: Parkell IC system[1], APM-Sterngold Plastic[2], Stutz Pivot[3], Ney[4], Para-Post[5].

To assure more accurate parallelism of the prepared canals, follow this procedure:

1. Select an abutment approximately in the middle of the other abutments.

2. Use the special sizing drill to prepare a canal in this root.

3. Place a post into this drilled root.

4. Drill all other canals using this post as a guide (Fig. 9-1).

Copings with customized dowels can also be used with some success. Generally, the root canal is enlarged with a tapered diamond bur. Impression material is then injected into the canal preparation to produce a removable die with the prepared dowel recess. Wax is flowed into this recess to form a wax post as part of the coping pattern to fabricate a casting with a customized gold post.

Parallel Canal Preparations Using An Intraoral Paralleling Device

The retention provided by a parallel-walled post such as the Whaledent Para-Post is superior to that provided by a tapered post. But it is difficult to accurately prepare, freehand, numerous parallel canals for parallel-walled dowels. A special intraoral paralleling device should be used (Figs. 9-2a and b) to drill these parallel canals. The jig must be stabilized in the mouth with a special template.

The Para-Post System for Parallel Canal Preparations

For this technique, the Para-Max intraoral parallator[1] is used to prepare parallel post canals or parallel pin holes intraorally. The Para-Post pre-sized drills are used to prepare the canal to receive pre-sized posts or pins.

Basic Materials for Para-Post Dowels and Pin Retention (Fig. 9-3)

1. Drills: Color-coded sized drills are available in three basic gauges for drilling sized holes; red (1.25 mm), black (1.50 mm), and green (1.75 mm). Smaller drills (0.036 and 0.040) are available for use with very narrow roots.

2. Posts: Four different types of posts are available: a) aluminium, b) stainless steel, c) gold, and d) plastic (smooth-walled and threaded).

The posts are parallel-walled and correspond to the diameter and shape of the drills used. The plastic and aluminum posts are color-coded to match the specific colored drill (corresponding diameter). The plastic posts become the dowel pattern. In addition, the smooth-walled plastic posts can also be used as the impression posts. The gold posts become an integral part of the wax pattern for a direct casting technique. The steel and aluminum posts are excellent for use with temporary resin crowns. The aluminum posts can also be used as impression posts.

3. CI Post drills[2]: The drills with this system have longer shafts than the Para-Post drills (Fig. 9-4). They therefore can be used with the Para-Max parallator to drill the initial canal preparation.

4. The Para-Max parallator is used to drill parallel post and parallel pin canals.

[1] Parkell Products Co., Farmingdale, N.Y.
[2] APM-Sterngold, San Mateo, Calif.
[3] APM-Sterngold, San Mateo, Calif.
[4] Ney, Bloomfield, Conn.
[5] Whaledent International, New York, N.Y.

[1] Whaledent International, New York, N.Y.
[2] Parkell Products Co., Farmingdale, N.Y.

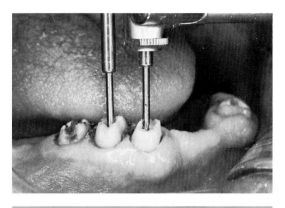

Fig. 9-1 "Free-hand" drilling of parallel canals for dowels with a tapered drill system. A centrally located root is prepared first and fitted with a dowel. The other canals are prepared by paralleling the drill to the inserted dowel.

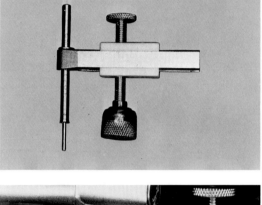

Fig. 9-2a The Para-Max is a special intraoral device for drilling parallel holes. It has a removable base (that is secured to a baseplate) connected to the vertical arm with a ball joint. This ball (and paralleler) joint is locked into position with the locking nut. The sliding horizontal arm houses the bushing that guides the drill while parallel holes are prepared.

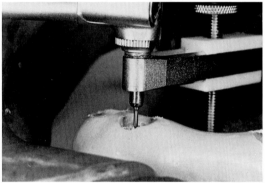

Fig. 9-2b The Para-Max is secured to a baseplate on a diagnostic cast. The baseplate is used to stabilize the jig in the mouth while drilling parallel holes.

Pin Materials (Fig. 9-5)

The Para-Post system also consists of a series of techniques for preparing parallel pin canals. They may utilize the template mounted Para-Max jig for preparing the parallel pin canals in multiple abutments, or, by using a special jig, to prepare pin canals parallel to a previously prepared dowel canal.

1. Three different kinds of pins are available: a) plastic, b) platinum-iridium, c) aluminum. The plastic pin is used as an impression pin or for patterns to produce castings with cast pins. The platinum-

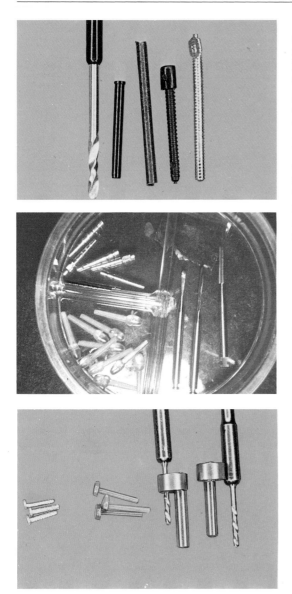

Fig. 9-3 An example of the basic Para-Post drill system (from left to right) consists of color-coded drill that prepare a sized canal (available in three sizes: red - 0.050, black - 0.060, green - 0.070), matching sized color-coded aluminum post used as dowel support for temporary crown, or as an impression post, sized color-coded plastic posts used as the casting pattern (or the impression posts).
These plastic patterns are available as threaded or non-threaded. The authors have found that the aluminum post diameter is generally smaller than the corresponding resin dowel. Therefore the resin dowel generally will not fit into its die recess. It is necessary to reduce the diameter of the resin dowel patterns until they do fit.

Fig. 9-4 CI drill and dowel post pattern system. The CI drill has a longer shaft than the Para-Post drill so it can be used to drill parallel dowel preparations when used with the Para-Max (the manufacturer plans to manufacture long shafted Para-Post drills).

Fig. 9-5 Instruments for making pin holes, from left to right, flat-headed nylon bristles used as impression pins (they may also be used as patterns for cast pins); aluminum pins for retaining temporary crowns; flat-headed platinum-iridium pins become an integral part of the pattern and casting; a special pin jig used to help prepare pin canals parallel to a previously prepared dowel canal, and a special pin drill.

iridium pins become an integral part of the wax pattern/and casting. The aluminum pins are used with temporary crowns for added retention.

2. A paralleling pin jig: This jig (available in three sizes corresponding to the three drill sizes), has a long shaft that matches the size of the post drill used. It has a disc with perforations 0.7 mm in diameter to match the 0.7 mm pin drill. The shaft of this jig is then inserted into a previously drilled canal; a pin drill is inserted into the jig pin holes to drill pin canals parallel to the previously drilled dowel canal.

3. An 0.7 mm pin drill: This drill is inserted through the jig holes to drill parallel canals to receive a 0.027 pin.

Para-Post Procedure for Parallel Post Canals

Follow these techniques to produce parallel post (or pin) holes in multiple abutments:

1. Prepare a study cast on which to fabricate an acrylic template (Fig. 9-6a).
2. Remove any teeth from the cast that are to be extracted.
3. Shorten the retained abutments on the cast to the approximate prepared length.
4. Fabricate an acrylic template covering the edentulous ridge and shortened abutments. Use self-curing resin or the vacuum-forming technique to fabricate this template (Fig. 9-6b).
5. Attach the Para-Max jig with auto-polymerizing resin to the template (Fig.9-6c).
6. Align the jig to drill holes to a common path of insertion (Fig. 9-6d).
7. The template must be stabilized on the abutments by relining the tissue side of the template with auto-polymerizing resin over these abutments.
8. Remove sufficient acrylic over each abutment to expose the surface of each root to receive the canal drill, and/or pin drills.
9. Stabilize the template jig in the mouth while drilling.
10. The canals are now drilled parallel to each other (Fig. 9-7). Note! Use a CI sizing reamer in the jig to drill the initial parallel post canals. The object is to drill parallel-walled post holes to receive the Para-Post dowels. However, the post drills supplied with the Para-Post system have a short shaft (longer shafted drills may be made available by the manufacturer). They, therefore, cannot be used with the Para-Max jig to drill post holes parallel to each other. Since the CI drills do have a longer shaft (and fit the Para-Max bushing) they are used instead to prepare these initial parallel canals. However, CI drills create a tapered canal that must be sized to accept a parallel-walled post. (The tapered canal will be sized with a Para-Post drill.)
11. Remove the jig from the mouth.
12. Now use the desired Para-Post drill and size each tapered post canal "free-hand" to receive the parallel-post impression post (Fig. 9-8).
13. Finally enlarge the occlusal opening of the post canal with a number six or eight round bur to half the depth of the bur head. This gives added strength to the casting (Fig. 9-9).
14. All canals are now parallel and will receive the Para-Post impression posts (Fig. 9-10).

Parallel pin holes can be drilled into each root with the same jig using appropriate twist drills. This will provide for a combination post and pin-retained coping (Figs. 9-11a and b).

Other Post Systems

Limitations of prefabricated plastic post systems, such as casting fit, can be eliminated by using prefabricated metal dowels. Dowel systems such as the Stutz Pivot[1] and

[1] APM-Sterngold, San Mateo, Calif.

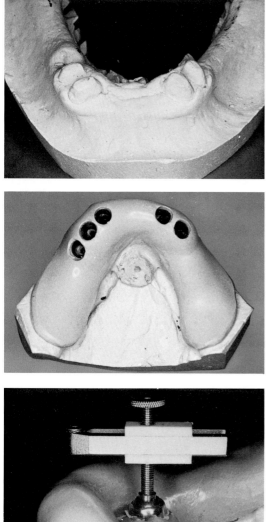

Fig. 9-6a Study cast prepared for fabrication of a resin template. The abutment teeth are shortened on the cast to the approximate level to be prepared in the mouth. The teeth to be removed are cut from the cast.

Fig. 9-6b Vacuum-formed, or auto-polymerized resin template fabricated on the prepared cast. For the lower template construct a small lingual table to receive the Para-Max base. Note the holes cut over the abutment teeth through which the drills must pass.

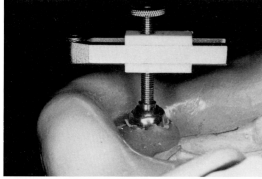

Fig. 9-6c Para-Max jig secured to the template. The jig must be mounted as far apically on the template as possible. This is necessary so that when post or pin drills are inserted through the jig bushing, they will reach the root surface with sufficient length for canal preparations.

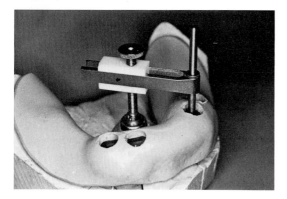

Fig. 9-6d The jig should be oriented so that a common drilling path is acceptable for all roots. This "leveling" can be done on the casts with a special paralleling rod.

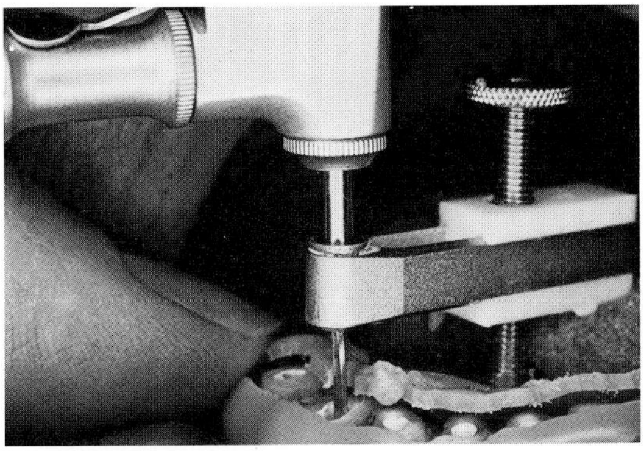

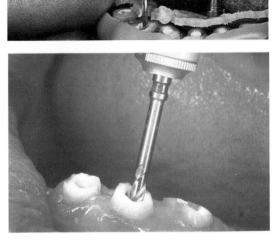

Fig. 9-7   The template is stabilized as the drill is passed through the jig bushing and into the root. The initial parallel canal preparations are first prepared with a CI drill (Note! A long shafted Para-Post drill that can be used to prepare this initial canal will be manufactured by Whaledent). If tapered dowel are desired these preparations need no further sizing.

Fig. 9-8   The tapered canal preparation drilled with the CI drill is now sized with the desired Para-Post drill.

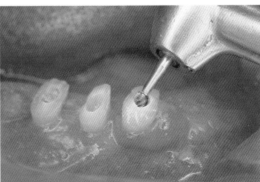

Fig. 9-9   The dowel preparation opening is enlarged with a number six or eight bur drilled half the diameter of the bur. This enlarged area provides for added thickness and strength here for the cast dowel. Use the number six bur for smaller dowel preparations.

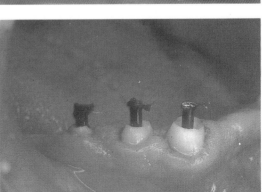

Fig. 9-10   Impression posts in the prepared canals prior to taking the impression. The nylon post patterns or aluminum posts can be used for this purpose. When the nylon posts are used, they should be shortened and their tops flattened with a hot instrument.

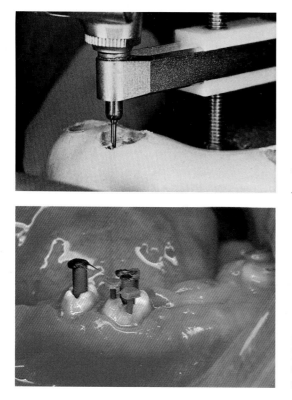

Fig. 9-11a Pin holes were prepared parallel to the post holes using the same template-mounted jig.

Fig. 9-11b Impression posts and pins were inserted into these preparations. The resultant casting will have a cast post and parallel pins for added retention.

Schenker Stepped Dowel[1], utilize special sizing drills and matching metal posts for accuracy of fit. Although metal posts can be notched slightly to provide a mechanical lock, there is a metallurgical bond between the post and the gold casting. It is the authors' experience that breakage of dowels, whether cast or prefabricated, is not a problem. The cast dowels are just as successful as the prefabricated types.

Stutz Pivot[1] (Fig. 9-12)

This tapered post system consists of sized drills used to prepare a single hole into the root. A hollow, silver shell is cemented permanently into the prepared root canal cavity with a seating tool. The metal post is insert-ed into the cemented shell to act as the impression post as well as the final dowel for the coping. The coping pattern is waxed to the metal post and cast for a metallurgical bond. For added strength the occlusal of the prepared post hole is shaped with a number six or eight bur to provide added thickness of gold here for more secure retention of the post.

Schenker Stepped Pivot[1] (Fig. 9-13)

This prefabricated metal post system has a stepped parallel-walled form in two different diameters for maximum retention. This design provides excellent retention for most short copings. The occlusal portion of the canal preparation should also be enlarged

[1] APM-Sterngold, San Mateo, Calif.

[1] APM-Sterngold, San Mateo, Calif.

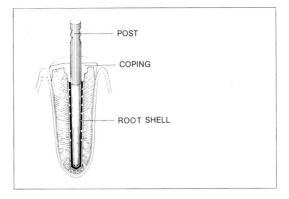

Fig. 9-12 Stutz pivot dowel system consists of a silver shell cemented into a prepared and sized canal; the dowel that becomes part of the coping fits into this cemented shell.

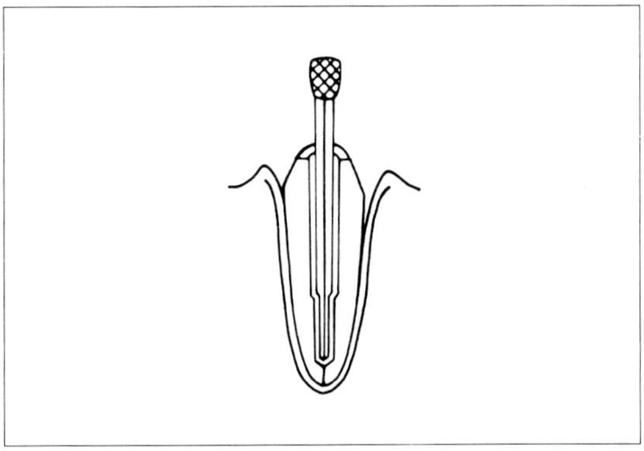

Fig. 9-13 The Schenker, a stepped parallel-walled dowel, increases the retention of the dowel coping and the root preparation. It is available in a large and a smaller size. The smaller end portion fits conveniently into the narrow root end.

with a round bur to provide added thickness of gold to provide a secure lock and bond to the post.

Parallel Pins

Condition of Teeth

Often the roots of abutment teeth are too short or divergent for effective post retention. Parallel pins for coping retention may be the only solution for this problem. For parallel pin retention the following is a suggested technique:

Parallel Pin Technique

1. Fabricate an acrylic template to secure and position the Para-Max jig similar to that discussed earlier (see Fig. 9-6c).

2. With a number two bur, drill small depressions into the root surfaces to receive the pin drill.

3. While stabilizing the Para-Max jig, insert the pin drill through the jig bushing and drill pin holes parallel to each other (Fig. 9-11a).

4. After all pin holes are prepared, insert the flat-head plastic impression pins (Fig. 9-14).

5. Take an impression of the prepared abutments, to produce a cast with removable dies (Fig. 9-15a). The impression pins are removed to provide holes to receive the metal pins.

6. Insert flat-headed platinum-iridium pins into the pin holes of each die (Fig. 9-15b). These pins are incorporated into the wax coping pattern (Fig. 9-15c). They then become an integral part of the metal casting (Fig. 9-15d).

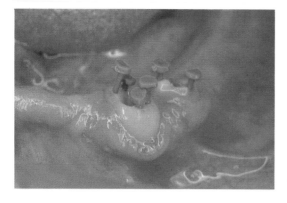

Fig. 9-14 Flat-headed nylon bristles inserted into the parallel pin holes. These impression pins are removed with the impression.

Post-Pin Retention

Probably the best method for effective coping retention is the post and pin combination (Fig. 9-16). This combination is useful where there is room for only a short three to four millimeter post; pins are added (in addition to the short post) for improved retention.

Several different techniques may be used depending on whether copings are a) to be splinted together – in this case all pin holes in all roots must be parallel to each other; or b) whether the copings are to be used singularly (in this case only the pin holes in each root must be parallel to each other).

With Splinted Copings

As mentioned earlier, when copings are to be splinted together, all post and pin holes must be drilled parallel to each other. This is easily accomplished with the same template and jig used to prepare the parallel post canals (see Figs. 9-6 and 9-7). Simply use an appropriate pin drill and make parallel pin holes where needed (see Fig. 9-11a). Now the root will have a post canal and parallel pin holes. Before the impression is taken, insert the impression post and nylon impression pins (see Fig. 9-11b). The prepared removable dies are then fitted with plastic post patterns and flat-headed platinum-iridium pins to be incorporated into the wax pattern to become the casting with a cast dowel and metal pins for retention.

With Separate Single Copings

When single copings are cemented on separate abutments, parallelism between abutments is not important.

The Para-Post system also lends itself to the fabrication of such post-pin retained copings for individual non-splinted abutments using a special parallel-pin jig (see Fig. 9-5).

Parallel post and pin canals are prepared in this manner:

1. First, prepare a post hole in the root canal with the desired size Para-Post drill (Fig. 9-17a).
2. Insert the special jig into the prepared canal (Fig. 9-17b).
3. Insert the pin drill through the jig holes and drill parallel pin holes directly into the root (Fig. 9-17c).
4. After the preparations are completed, insert the nylon impression posts and pin bristles into the prepared canals (Fig. 9-17d). The impression is taken to obtain a cast with removable dies to fabricate castings with a single post and pins parallel to each other (Figs. 9-16 and 9-17e).

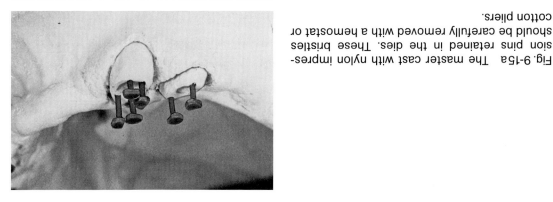

Fig. 9-15a The master cast with nylon impression pins retained in the dies. These bristles should be carefully removed with a hemostat or cotton pliers.

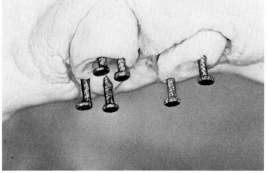

Fig. 9-15b Appropriate size (0.7 mm) platinum-iridium pins replace the nylon bristles. These metal pins should fit into the pin canals without being forced. They become an integral part of the coping pattern.

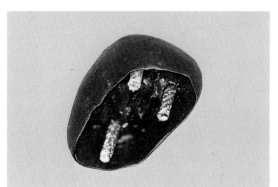

Fig. 9-15c A wax coping pattern with the platinum-iridium pins incorporated in the wax-up.

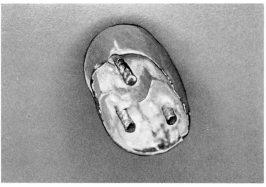

Fig. 9-15d A parallel pin coping with platinum-iridium pins incorporated into the casting. The parallel pin adds excellent retention with short-walled abutments.

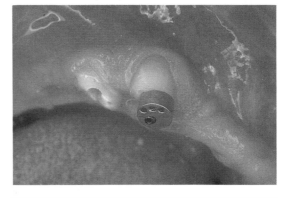

Fig. 9-17c   The twist drill is inserted through the bushings and holes drilled parallel to the dowel canal. The jig acts as a paralleling device.

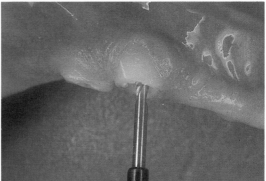

Fig. 9-17b   A pin jig inserted into the prepared dowel canal. Select the proper size jig to match the drilled hole.

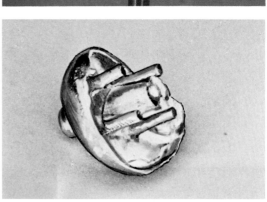

Fig. 9-17a   Abutment prepared with pin canals parallel to a dowel preparation. A parallel-walled dowel canal prepared with a Para-Post drill.

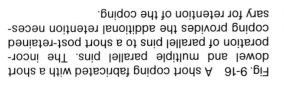

Fig. 9-16   A short coping fabricated with a short dowel and multiple parallel pins. The incorporation of parallel pins to a short post-retained coping provides the additional retention necessary for retention of the coping.

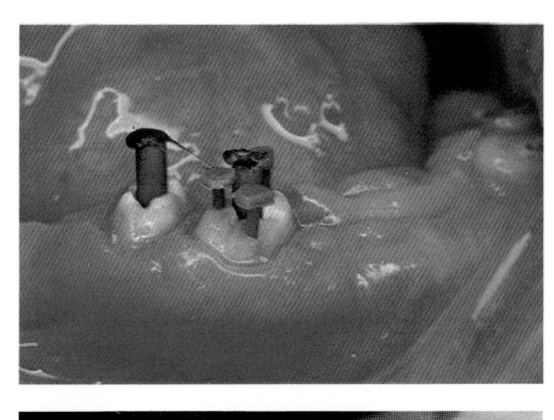

Fig. 9-17 d   The impression pins and dowels in position for the impression of the abutments.

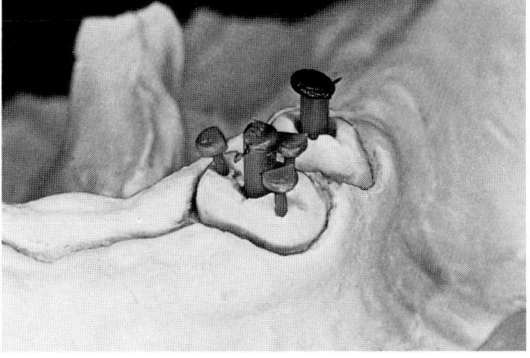

Fig. 9-17 e   The master cast with the impression pins and plastic dowel incorporated in the dies. The nylon pins are replaced with metal pins.

Chapter 10

Impressions – Casts – Occlusal Registration

Impressions

Impressions for abutment preparations and removable prosthetic appliances vary with an operator's preference and experience. Techniques proven successful for routine crown and bridge, removable partial and complete denture prosthetics should be continued.

When taking impressions for an overdenture prosthesis, not only must you be concerned with an accurate impression of the abutment teeth, but also the denture-bearing mucosa. A correctly extended muscle-trimmed impression with a customized tray is a prerequisite for a satisfactory overdenture. However, it is often difficult to obtain an accurate recording of the abutment teeth and tissue areas with the same impression. In addition, the simple procedure of sawing and trimming of dies will destroy the accuracy of the master cast for overlay prosthesis fabrication. The authors feel that best results are obtained when separate impressions are taken for the copings and the overdenture.

The abutment impression is taken just for fabrication of the copings and for attachment assembly. An impression for the overlay prosthesis is taken of the tissue-bearing mucosa with the copings cemented (temporarily or permanently) or the substructure is "pulled" with this impression. Use of elastic or rigid impression materials may vary to produce some of these working casts:

1. Casts for fabrication of the copings and attachment assembly only (elastic).
2. Cast for fabrication of the coping and overdenture (elastic).
3. Cast of the substructure cemented on the abutments for fabrication of the overdenture (elastic).
4. Cast of the substructure cemented on abutments with a special transfer male technique (this procedure to be discussed thoroughly later in the text) (elastic).
5. Cast with the substructure "pulled" with the impression (elastic or rigid).

Custom Trays

Generally, abutment preparations can be accurately recorded with elastic impression materials using stock trays. However, it is difficult to stabilize the tray and impression material, since reduction of the clinical crowns has eliminated their supporting feature. A custom tray is often a solution to this problem.

Custom trays can be fabricated of vacuum-formed materials, or, as described here, of auto-polymerizing resin.

1. Prepare the cast for fabrication of the tray. The abutments on the cast must be reduced as those in the mouth. Remove the teeth on the cast of those to be extracted.

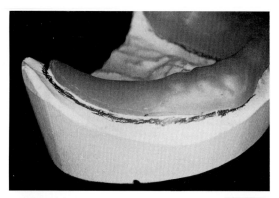

Figs. 10-1a to f   A customized tray fabricated on the diagnostic cast. Use a vacuum-forming technique or, as shown here, auto-polymerizing tray material.

Fig. 10-1a   Adapt one layer of baseplate wax 2-3 millimeters short of the muscle attachment outlined on the cast.

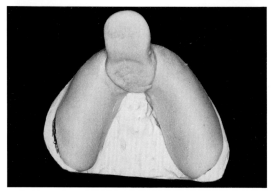

Fig. 10-1b   Adapt doughy tray material over the wax spacer beyond the edges of the wax. A handle should be added for ease of impression taking.

2. Outline the peripheral border (the muscle attachment area) on the cast.
3. Adapt a single thickness of baseplate wax to several millimeters short of this outline (Fig. 10-1a). Use two thicknesses of damp asbestos if a vacuum-formed tray is to be constructed.
4. Adapt a doughy pad of tray resin over the wax spacer. Form a handle on the tray (Fig. 10-1b).
5. Remove the cured tray from the cast, shape and reduce its flanges to the wax spacer outline (Fig. 10-1c).
6. Remove all baseplate wax except in those areas that will act as stops when taking an impression. These stops should be located in the posterior areas and one in the anterior area, but not over the abutments (Fig. 10-1d).
7. Drill holes in the tray over the abutments to expose the root surfaces when the tray is inserted. The tray must be modified in this manner if the abutments were prepared for dowel-post or pin retained copings. The impression tray must not press on the extruding impression posts, pins, or attachments (Fig. 10-1e).
8. Add soft modeling compound to the tray margin, temper in warm water, insert into the mouth and muscle-trim the compound.
   Muscle-trimming is not necessary if the impression is to record just the abutment preparation for coping fabrication (Fig. 10-1f).
9. Scrape away approximately one to two millimeters of the peripheral compound to provide space for the impression material.
10. Paint the tissue area of the tray with an adhesive. It is now ready for taking a muscle-trimmed impression.

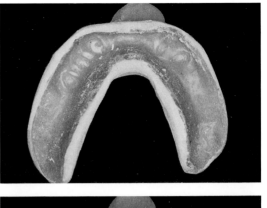

Fig. 10-1c Remove the hardened tray and trim the flange to the edge of the wax spacer.

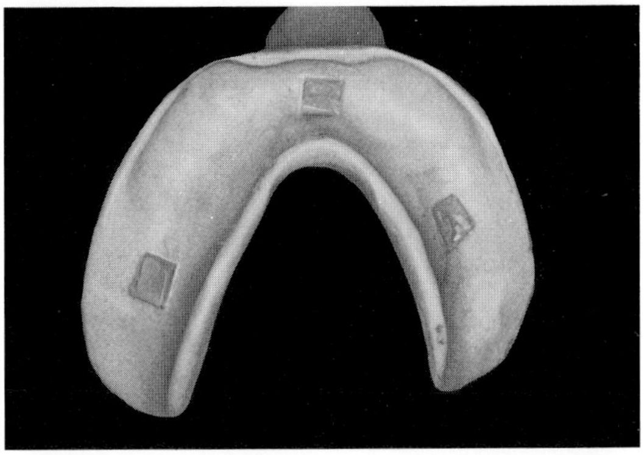

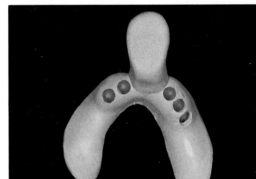

Fig. 10-1d Remove the wax spacer leaving three small squares, as shown here, to act as stops.

Fig. 10-1e Holes were drilled over the abutments to prevent dislodgement or misalignment of the post, pins or attachments.

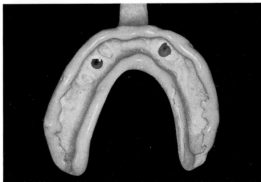

Fig. 10-1f The custom tray muscle-trimmed for an accurate impression of the soft-tissue attachment areas.

Abutment Impressions and Casts

Accurate impressions of the abutments should be taken with the materials of the operator's choice. The impression of the abutments can be taken with hydrocolloid, rubber base, polyether, or silicone impression materials. The impression is treated according to customary laboratory procedures to produce the master cast with removable dies for coping fabrication and attachment assembly.

The accuracy of the impression, dies and finished copings cannot be any better than marginal exposure of the preparation. But it is of the utmost importance that the gingival tissues receive minimal trauma. To expose this margin, use a straight electrosurgery needle held approximately fifteen degrees away from the cavo-surface bevel and slightly below the crest of the gingiva. Pass this needle smoothly around the entire periphery without causing extensive tissue damage of the preparation, with the current set for moderate cutting action (Fig. 10-2). Also remove any excess fibrous tissue on the ridge or near the proximal surface of the abutments.

Next, irrigate the gingival crevice area with hydrogen peroxide to remove any debris produced by the electrosurgical procedure. If bleeding is present, inject a small drop of Xylocaine[1] with epinephrine into the more fibrous proximal tissue for its hemostasis effect. Be prepared to take the impression immediately before bleeding resumes. If bleeding persists, the gingiva can be gently packed with some form of astringent string. Load the impression tray with accurately proportioned heavy body material and the syringe with light body injectable material. Thoroughly inject the light body material into the gingival crevice, around each abutment tooth and around the impression posts and pins. Carefully press down on all posts or pins, making certain that they are completely inserted into the roots.

Carefully insert the loaded tray into position. If the copings will be dowel-retained, the impression posts should pass through the opening prepared in the tray but still covered with impression material. If the impression is used to produce a cast for the overdenture fabrication in addition to copings, it must be muscle-trimmed immediately. After the muscle-trimming procedure, hold the impression tray steady in this position to accurately record the abutment teeth without distortion. Remove the set impression, clean it thoroughly and carefully examine it for accuracy. It can now be poured to produce a cast with removable dies.

Before pouring the impression, coat the exposed portion of each post with a very thin film of silicone material, such as Masque[1] (Fig. 10-3). This facilitates the release of the impression posts with less danger of fracturing the stone dies. Pour the impression with appropriate die material and then a stone base material to produce a master cast with removable dies.

If the impression includes posts, before separating the impression from the set cast, carefully remove all impression material over the dies exposing the locked-in impression post (Fig. 10-4). Gently clasp each post with a narrow-beaked hemostat and carefully rotate and tease it out (Fig. 10-5). Removing the model from the impression with the posts still in place may break the dies and destroy the master cast. But there is no such danger with nylon pin bristles. The cast can now be removed from the impression.

When this master cast is to be used for fabrication of the overdenture as well as the copings, duplicate the cast in refractory material before sawing and trimming the dies. The metal reinforcement framework for this overdenture can then be fabricated on this refractory cast. The framework should

[1] Astra Pharmaceuticals, Inc.

[1] Harry J. Bosworth Co., Chicago

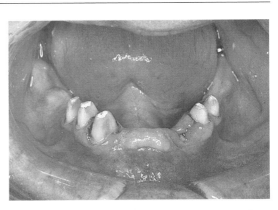

Fig. 10-2 A thin electrosurgery needle was used carefully to expose the prepared margin prior to impression taking. Judicious use of the electrosurgery needle is important to avoid damage to the tissues.

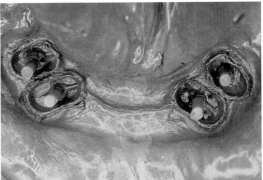

Fig. 10-3 Exposed impression posts extending out of the impression material should be carefully painted with a thin layer of silicone. This aids in their removal from the dies.

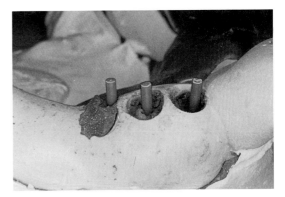

Fig. 10-4 The impression is poured with stone and after the stone has hardened sufficiently, impression material is removed carefully from over the abutment areas to expose the impression posts. Damage to the dies may occur if the impression is removed before prior removal of the impression material.

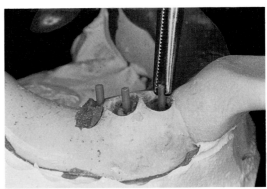

Fig. 10-5 The impression post is removed by carefully rotating the post with a hemostat. Exert a straight upward pressure to avoid breaking the die.

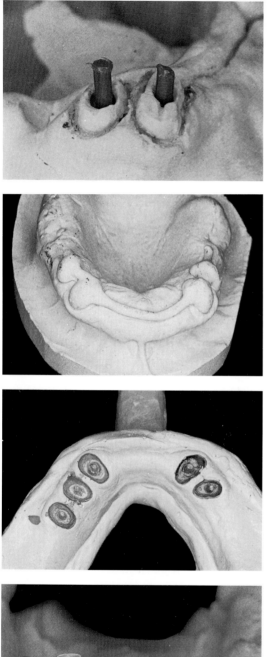

Fig. 10-6   Master cast removed from the impression and the dowel patterns are returned to their original position on the trimmed dies.

Fig. 10-7   A master cast fabricated from an impression taken with the substructure cemented on the abutments. This is the recommended procedure when the substructure may be single copings or coping and some bar combinations. Stone reproduction of most stud attachments would have inadequate strength for withstanding the overdenture fabrication techniques. In this situation, special transfer attachment components are used when stud-copings are cemented on their abutments.

Fig. 10-8   Coping substructure pulled with a ZOE impression taken for fabrication of the overdenture. Before the impression is poured with stone, cover the posts or any exposed pins with wax. There will be less danger of damaging these posts and pins when the substructure is removed from the cast after overdenture fabrication.

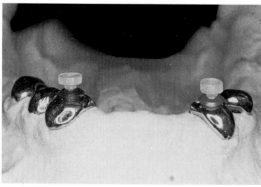

Fig. 10-9   A master cast for the fabrication of the overdenture with the metal substructure an integral part of the cast. This is especially recommended when attachments such as studs cannot be duplicated in stone to withstand the overdenture fabrication techniques, or when transfer attachment components are not used.

be designed to cover or compensate for the sawing and die-ditching procedure.

The dies can be trimmed and ditched for waxing of the copings. The plastic dowel pattern can be repositioned into the dies, and any nylon pin bristles replaced with platinum-iridium pins (Fig. 10-6). One will notice that the plastic dowel patterns may fit too tightly which would make removal of the wax pattern difficult. The diameter of these dowel patterns should be reduced slightly with a sharp knife before inserting them into the die recess.

Overdenture Impressions and Casts

A custom tray should be used to take a muscle-trimmed impression for fabrication of the overdenture. An elastic or rigid material may be used, depending on the specific situation. An elastic impression must be used if the substructure is cemented on the abutments and cannot be pulled with the impression although it can also be used when the substructure is pulled. Rigid impression materials may be used only when the substructure is pulled. Cementing the substructure permanently has its advantages, however. This eliminates any error in coping fit and cementation. This simple procedure solves one of the problem areas of overdenture prosthetics and is highly recommended.

Thus, the recommended casts for overdenture fabrication may be reproductions of the denture-bearing mucosa and –

1. the substructure cemented on the abutments,

2. the substructure "pulled" with the impression,

3. the substructure cemented on the abutments using a male transfer technique (this technique will be described more thoroughly later in the text when discussing specific attachments).

Substructure Cemented on Abutments

Metal substructures such as simple primary copings or copings with bar attachments, are easily duplicated in stone (Fig. 10-7). Plaster reproductions of such copings and bar attachments have sufficient bulk and strength to withstand the stresses of overdenture fabrication techniques. If possible, it is always advisable to cement the substructure on the abutments. Then simply take a muscle-trimmed master impression with an elastic impression material to record the denture-supporting tissues and the cemented substructure. This resultant cast is used for the overdenture fabrication.

Casts with Substructure "Pulled" with Impression

Often the coping substructure will have narrow stud-like attachments that cannot be duplicated in stone to withstand overdenture fabricating techniques.

This situation can be managed by "pulling" the substructure with the master impression (Fig. 10-8). The substructure thus becomes an integral part of the master cast when the impression is poured (Fig. 10-9). Here, a wider selection of impression materials is applicable: elastic materials, ZOE paste, impression plaster, Hydrocast, etc.).

Since many copings have dowel or pin retention, these retentive features must be covered with a thin layer of wax before the impression is poured. Now the copings are more easily removed from the cast after overdenture fabrication.

Casts with Substructure Cemented Using Transfer Males

If a substructure with stud attachments has been cemented, this situation can be managed by using special transfer males that become an integral part of the cast. This is accomplished in this manner (covered in greater detail later in the text on specific attachments).

1. Place the females on the males in the mouth.
2. The females can be provided with a resin cap to provide a definite "lock" in the impression material.
3. Take a muscle-trimmed impression with an elastic impression material which will withdraw the female.
4. Place special transfer males into the females.
5. Pour the impression with model stone to produce a cast with the male studs in the exact location as in the mouth.
6. This cast is now used for fabrication of the overdenture (Fig. 10-10).

Cast Orientation

An overdenture's occlusal relationship, in harmony during all functional movements of the mandible, is just as important for success as with other restorative procedures. One's technique for recording these occlusal relationships proven successful for partial and complete denture prosthodontics should be continued, or modified whenever desirable. Accurate records must be used to mount the master casts on an appropriate articulator of the dentist's choice.

Articulation of Casts for Coping Fabrication and Attachments

Accurate occlusal records and orientation of master casts for coping fabrication is not as critical as that for fabrication of the overdenture. Generally, overdenture copings are short and not fabricated in occlusion with the opposing dentition. Since a favorable crown-root ratio is always desirable, sufficient intraocclusal space is generally present. However, accurate occlusal records and cast orientation are extremely important if the primary copings are fitted with porcelain-to-metal secondary copings in occlusal contact with the opposing dentition.

When the intraocclusal space is limited, accurately oriented casts are important for attachment selection and placement. Often attachments with minimum vertical height must be selected in close bite situations.

Orientation of Casts for Overdenture Fabrication

Of course, accurately mounted master casts for overdenture fabrication are particularly important. However, accurate occlusal records are impossible without well-fitting record bases.

These record bases may be wax, shellac, heat cured or auto-polymerizing resin, or the overdenture framework fitted with attachments. The authors recommend using "stabilized" auto-polymerizing or heat-cured resin record bases or the overdenture framework, particularly when they are fitted with the attachments when these are used.

Record Bases

Stabilized Wax or Shellac Record Bases

The disadvantage of wax and shellac bases is their lack of rigidity and adaptation to the tissue. Their fit can be overcome by stabilizing the bases with materials such as zinc oxide impression material. However, they still lack rigidity, particularly for use with attachments for retention.

Resin Bases

An excellent record base may be fabricated of auto-polymerizing or heat-cured resin. An auto-polymerizing base may be made by placing a doughy mix of auto-polymerizing resin in a matrix (wax or shellac) and then adapting it to a duplicated cast.

Or, a record base may be made by a "sprinkled" technique requiring repeated application of powder and then liquid. A superior heat-cure resin base is made similar to the technique for complete denture fabrication (Fig. 10-11). The base plate is waxed on the cast, flasked, packed, cured and finished.

Because the resin base is very rigid, all undercuts must be relieved from inside the denture base; otherwise, the base will be prevented from fitting on the cast. The accuracy of these bases for recording occlusal relationships can be improved by adding the female (or male) component of the attachment. Now the bases, with their occlusal rims, will be root-retained and supported.

Framework Record Bases

The overdenture framework makes an excellent record base, particularly when fitted with the removable attachment component and occlusal rims (see chapter 12 for a more thorough discussion of framework design, Fig. 10-12). If an all-metal saddle framework is used, simply secure the removable attachment component and occlusal rims and take the occlusal records. If the framework is fabricated with a retentive mesh for the resin denture base, it must be modified to fit the ridges in this manner: adapt a layer of foil to the ridge area; flow hot wax over the foil covering the retentive mesh. Now the attachment and wax rims can be added to take all necessary records. When used in this manner, the framework should be fabricated with knobs or ringlets especially designed for securing the removable attachment component (Figs. 10-13 and 10-14).

Occlusal Registration

These bases are used for taking occlusal records according to the dentist's preference, with wax occlusal rims using soft wax or plaster to record centric, intraoral or extraoral techniques.

Maxillary casts should always be oriented on an appropriate articulator with a face-bow transfer. The lower cast is then oriented to the upper with the above records.

The accuracy of these records may be verified with split-cast mounting or some centric check-point technique of the dentist's choice.

Functionally Generated Occlusal Technique

The attachment-retained and stabilized record bases lend themselves for fabricating functional occlusion in metal using the functionally generated path technique (FGP):

1. Lower dentition is restored (lower incisal length, posterior plane of occlusion, and cuspal inclination).
2. A special overdenture framework (Fig. 10-12) is fabricated with parallel posterior struts.
3. Upper anterior teeth are positioned for esthetics (Fig. 10-13).
4. Resin is added temporarily to the lingual surfaces of the upper anterior and adjusted for centric and anterior guidance (or the anterior teeth may be processed and adjusted for centric and anterior guidance).
5. A resin table is added posteriorly to vertical parallel posts on the specially fabricated framework. It must be clear occlusally (Fig. 10-14).
6. Soft wax[1] is added to occlusal table.
7. The patient's mandible is guided into intercuspal position and then moved through all excursions. (The lower cusps act as stylii, carving a mandibular functional record in wax (Fig. 10-15).
8. The attachment-retained framework is removed from the mouth and transferred to the master cast.

[1] J. F. Jelenko Co., New Rochelle, N.Y.

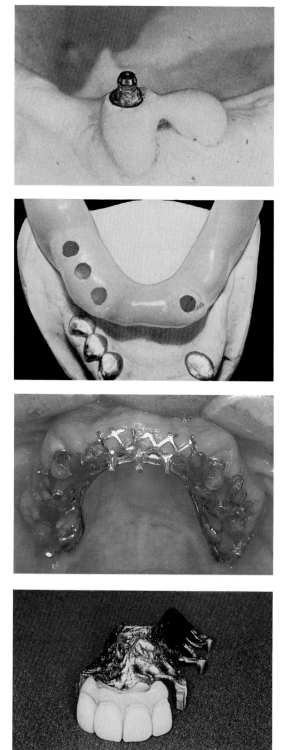

Fig. 10-10 A master cast, with transfer males, to be used for fabrication of the overdenture. The transfer males are an exact replica of the originals and in exactly the same position as in the mouth.

Fig. 10-11 Heat-cured resin record base fabricated for taking attachment-retained records. Holes were drilled through the base to receive the female attachment which will be locked to the base with resin.

Fig. 10-12 Overdenture framework to be used as an attachment fixation record base. The removable attachment component has been locked to the framework with resin. A wax occlusal rim is then added to the framework.

Fig. 10-13 Anterior teeth set up for esthetics and checked for occlusal accuracy. The anterior denture component can be processed, or resin added to the lingual surface. Centric occlusion and anterior guidance is developed in resin on the articulated casts and the occlusion is refined in the mouth.

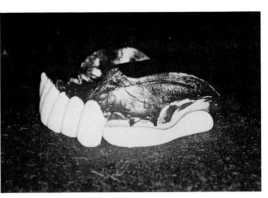

Fig. 10-14   A removable resin table is fabricated to fit over the special parallel studs. This table must be clear of the lower posterior teeth when the patient closes in centric.

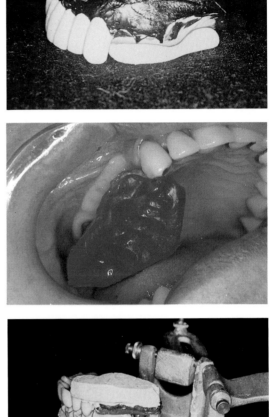

Fig. 10-15   A functionally generated occlusal record is taken as the mandible closes into centric and then moves through all functional excursions.

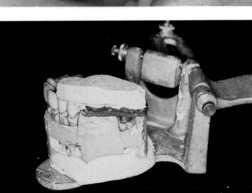

Fig. 10-16   The framework with the functional record is removed from the mouth, placed on the master cast and articulated to a Hanau twin-stage articulator.

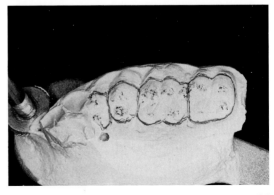

Fig. 10-17   Stone is poured into the functional record and articulated to the opposite member of the articulator. An opposite anatomical cast is also articulated to the functional core.

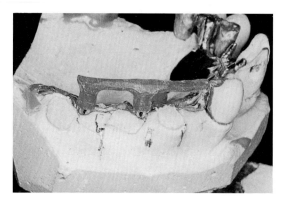

Fig. 10-18   A removable resin framework is fabricated to fit over the struts. The functional pattern will be waxed to this removable resin framework.

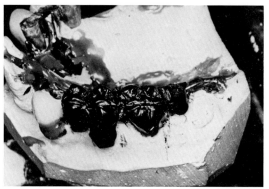

Fig. 10-19   The removable pattern is waxed to the stone core, producing functional occlusal anatomy; the pattern is reduced facially for a veneer to receive porcelain when cast.

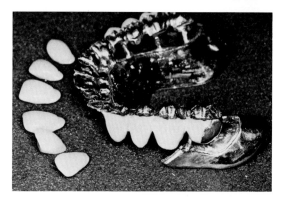

Fig. 10-20   Porcelain processed on the facial area of the functionally generated casting.

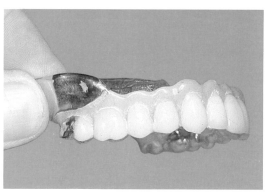

Fig. 10-21   The customized units are repositioned on the framework struts and locked in position when the overdenture denture base is processed.

9. A die stone is poured into the posterior functional record (as well as the anterior).

10. The master cast is mounted to the lower member of a Hanau twin-stage articulator[1].

11. The die stone core and an anatomical model are articulated to the opposite members of the articulator (Figs. 10-16 and 10-17).

12. The FGP record and resin table removed from the framework and a removable resin strut is fabricated to fit the parallel posts (Fig. 10-18).

13. Wax is added to the resin strut and horizontal bar, and porcelain veneer patterns are waxed to the FGP stone record. The occlusal anatomy of the restoration will be in harmony with mandibular movement if fabricated similar to techniques thoroughly described in other texts. The facial area of the removable wax pattern is carved as for maxillary posterior porcelain veneer restorations (Fig. 10-19).

14. The pattern is cast in a non-precious metal (or gold) that will receive porcelain (Fig. 10-20).

15. This separate restoration unit (with porcelain veneer added) is repositioned on the framework posts and locked into position when the denture base is processed (Fig. 10-21). Note! This wax pattern can be cast directly to the framework and porcelain added to the casting locked on the framework. However, this latter technique complicates the procedure since the framework must now be re-polished. The prior technique is preferred.

[1] Hanau Engineering Co., Inc., Buffalo, N.Y.

Chapter 11

Waxed Patterns and Coping Consideration

The sawed, trimmed and lubricated dies are used to develop wax patterns for accurately fitting copings. The finished casting will be no better than the quality of the wax pattern. The shape and contour of wax patterns will depend on its function and determined in part by the abutment preparations. Of course the preparation is determined by the type of coping selected. Therefore, a discussion of wax pattern form is really a review of the four basic coping designs: long, medium, medium-short and short (see chapter 4). This chapter will also discuss the effect of pattern design on esthetics, periodontal health, and relation of coping function to pattern design.

Coping Consideration

It is important to remember that wax patterns (and copings) must be designed for:

– Periodontal health
– Esthetics
– Stability and support
– Retention
– Use with stud attachments
– Use with bar attachments
– Use with auxiliary attachments

Coping Patterns for Periodontal Health

Periodontal health is of utmost importance with any form of crown and bridge prosthesis. When waxing patterns for copings, minimally-contoured crowns with good embrasures provide a healthy environment for long-range success of the overlay prosthesis. The copings should never be over-contoured with excessive undercuts (Fig. 11-1). Such over-contoured copings produce space between the coping, the overdenture, and the mucosa where gingival tissue will proliferate.

When several close short copings are connected together, it is often difficult to develop good embrasures. Here the pattern should extend slightly higher interproximally to allow room for good interproximal, facial and lingual embrasures (Fig. 11-2).

When these short copings are further apart, they can be connected with a short strut-like bar (Fig. 11-3). This bar should be in light contact with the gingival tissues along its length. Often, this strut may be placed slightly lingual, even positioned in slight depressions to allow room for the denture teeth set-up (Fig. 11-4).

Creating good embrasures is easier with long copings. When the abutments are close together, normal embrasures should be developed interproximally (Fig. 11-5a). When the abutments are slightly further apart, place a small connecting bar between the copings occlusally (Fig. 11-5b). If the copings are still further apart, drop the connecting bar to rest in light contact with the gingival tissues (Fig. 11-5c).

Where teeth have extensive bone loss facially or lingually, contour the pat-

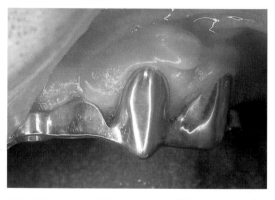

Fig. 11-1 Copings with well-developed contours and embrasures are important for maintenance of periodontal health. The copings tapered with a high interproximal connector, assuring an ideal gingival embrasure. A narrow connector facially-lingually helps to develop wide open facial and lingual embrasures.

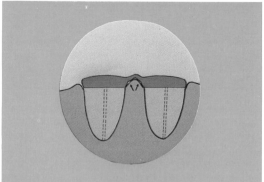

Fig. 11-2 Art sketch of two close, short coping patterns connected together. The patterns have a convex occlusal diaphragm. This surface follows closely the ridge contour. The short axial surfaces should have no undercuts. The interproximal connector is narrow facially-lingually and elevated occlusally. The elevated connector helps to develop good gingival, facial and lingual embrasures.

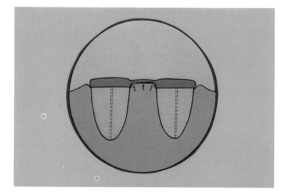

Fig. 11-3 Wax patterns for short copings farther apart and connected with a strut. The connecting bar is in light contact with the tissues. The proximal gingival area, where the bar connects the coping patterns, must have an open embrasure for the proximal tissues.

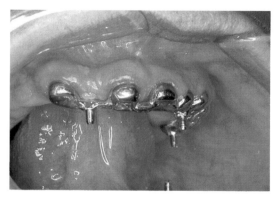

Fig. 11-4 A connecting strut placed in a lingual position between two copings.

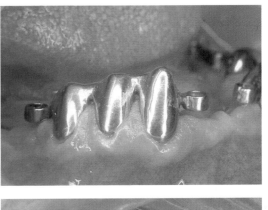

Fig. 11-5a Well-developed gingival, facial and lingual embrasure with tapered copings.

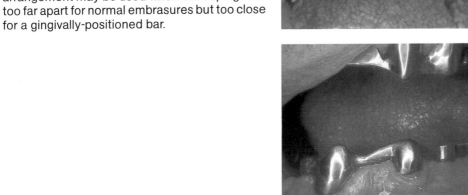

Fig. 11-5b Tapered long copings connected with an occlusally-positioned strut. Such an arrangement may be used when the copings are too far apart for normal embrasures but too close for a gingivally-positioned bar.

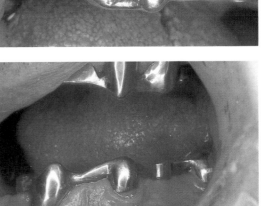

Fig. 11-5c Medium copings with the connecting strut in light contact with the alveolar ridge.

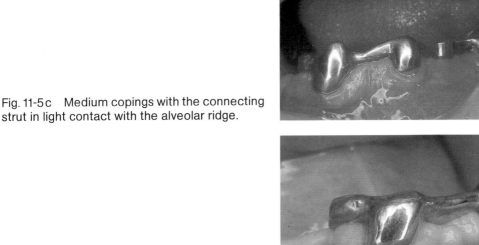

Fig. 11-5d Wax patterns should produce copings to compensate for the soft and bony tissue deformities. The coping is contoured into these areas to help maintain the health of the supporting tissues.

tern so that the copings fits into these deformities to compensate for the tissue loss. This helps to protect and maintain the health of the remaining tissues (Fig. 11-5d).

Coping Patterns for Esthetics

Esthetics is a major concern particularly in the upper anterior. Bulky copings interfere with the normal set-up of the denture teeth and cause cosmetic failure of the overdenture treatment. Therefore, short copings should closely follow the contour of the anterior alveolar ridge, being slightly flat occlusal-lingually to receive the stud attachments (see Fig. 4-6). Therefore anterior abutment teeth should be prepared to allow room for this low coping profile. Where long copings are used, maximum room should be left facially for set-up of teeth. The coping should taper (see Figs. 4-2a and b). Where a porcelain-to-metal secondary coping is to fit over the primary coping, the pattern should have a heavy shoulder (see Fig. 4-3). The shoulder margin should be even with the gingival crest. The rest of the coping should taper dramatically, particularly if an auxiliary form of retention is to be incorporated. If a plunger-type of attachment is to be used, at least one side (proximal preferable) should be flattened to receive a depression engaged by the plunger (see Fig. 4-1b).

Coping Patterns for Stability and Support

Patterns for copings designed simply to support the overdenture are very short, with a dome-like convex occlusal surface. This surface follows closely the contour of the alveolar ridge, approximately one to two mm above the ridge contour (Fig. 11-6).

When individual medium-short copings are designed to provide stability in addition to support, they are slightly longer, extending occlusally two to four mm. Their overall form is conical (Fig. 11-7).

Coping Patterns for Retention

As already discussed in chapter 4, long copings can provide retention through frictional contact with the proximal walls of the telescopic overdenture. However, all proximal walls need not be parallel. Only the gingival one-third to one-half of the proximal walls are semi-parallel (Fig. 11-8). Other surfaces taper occlusally. Similarly, there will be some parallelism to other copings in the same arch. Often just one proximal wall of each of several copings may be parallel. The facial and lingual surfaces taper along their entire length. The facial surface should taper more to the lingual to allow maximum room for set-up of anterior teeth.

When long primary copings function with secondary copings made of metal or of porcelain-to-metal, the primary copings should have a definite shoulder (Fig. 11-9). A heavy shoulder permits an accurate fit and room for the more bulky secondary coping. This makes it possible to develop a crown with normal contour and excellent cosmetics. The shoulder should not be below the gingiva, but even with the gingival margin for gingival health and appearance (Fig. 11-10).

Since metal-to-metal contact causes much wear, it is ill-advised to rely entirely on the parallelism of coping walls for retention. If no attachments are to be used, cut a small hole in the proximal surface of each secondary coping to allow room for processed acrylic resin. Now retention can be adjusted by replacing or relining the resin in this hole only.

Coping Patterns for Stud Attachments

Most stud attachments are designed for use with short copings. For these attachments

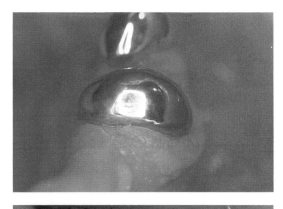

Fig. 11-6 A short coping designed for support. The contour conforms to the alveolar ridge one to two millimeters above the gingiva.

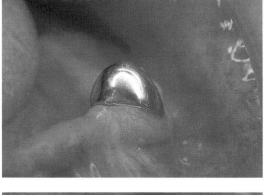

Fig. 11-7 Medium-short copings designed to provide support and stability for the overdenture. Its overall contour is conical in form.

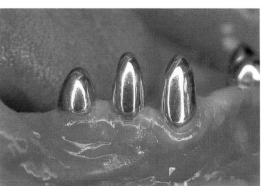

Fig. 11-8 Copings designed for retention. The gingival one-third to one-half of the proximal surfaces are closely parallel. The occlusal two-thirds to one-half is tapering. Note the coping on the left, designed only for support and stability.

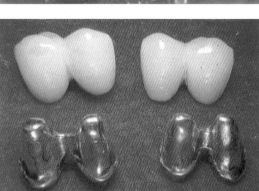

Fig. 11-9 Coping designed with a shoulder to receive a porcelain-to-metal secondary coping. The secondary coping will fit flush with the primary coping shoulder.

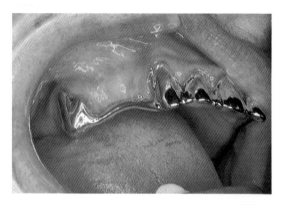

Fig. 11-10   The shoulder should be even with the gingival margin when the overdenture is inserted. This type of fit will not irritate the gingiva.

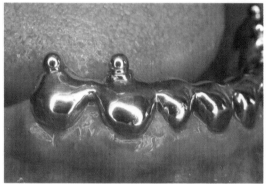

Fig. 11-11   Short copings designed to receive a stud attachment.

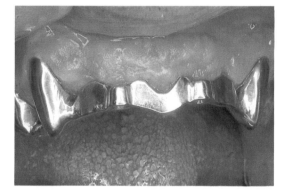

Fig. 11-12   Long copings designed for use with bar attachments should be very tapered. Retention is obtained with the bar attachment and not with coping parallelism.

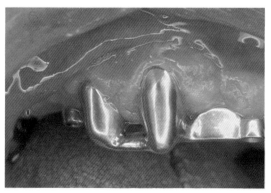

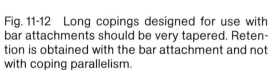

Fig. 11-13   Medium copings used in conjunction with a bar attachment. Such coping patterns must be very tapered and conical in form.

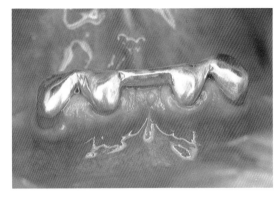

Fig. 11-14   Short copings used with bar attachments. The interproximal connectors should be elevated to provide a healthy environment for the gingiva.

the patterns for copings should be kept as close to the ridge as possible. A short coping should have a convex contour, closely following the contour of the alveolar ridge (Fig. 11-11). It is much less conical than copings designed for stability.

When the gingival margin is more or less uniform, the wax pattern should conform to the contour of the alveolar ridge. The diaphragm of the coping should be approximately 0.5-1 millimeter thick.

The diaphragm's strength is derived from the cross cut in the occlusal surface of the preparation and from the thickness at the opening of the dowel hole made by enlarging the occlusal opening of the canal with a number eight rounded bur.

Coping Patterns for Bar Attachments

Bar attachments can be used with all coping forms.

When long copings are to be used with bar attachments, the coping pattern should be very tapered. As the bar will retain the overdenture, the copings need not be designed for retention (Fig. 11-12). This extreme tapering form allows maximum room for set-up of denture teeth. Of course the preparations must be made with this in mind. Medium copings should also taper but be more conical or bullet-shaped than long copings (Fig. 11-13).

Short coping patterns for bar attachments are similar to short copings for stud attachments. However, the proximal surface connecting the bars should be elevated. This provides room for good embrasures at the bar-coping junction for periodontal health (Fig. 11-14).

Coping Patterns for Auxiliary Attachments[1]

Auxiliary attachments such as the plunger-type IC and Ipsoclip can be used with long or medium copings. The copings are similar to those used with bar attachments with one exception: they have a flattened surface with a small round depression the size of a number four bur to receive the spring-loaded plunger (see Fig. 4-1b).

Waxing Procedure

Fabricating a coping pattern is a simple procedure since there is no occlusal anatomy, or coronal contour important with routine restorative procedures. Most coping patterns are simple thimbles of wax adapted over the lubricated die.

These patterns can be made rapidly with various techniques, depending on the coping type:

[1] APM Sterngold, San Mateo, Calif.

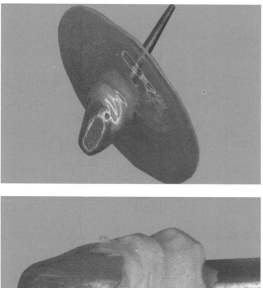

Fig. 11-15a Resin patterns vacuumed over the trimmed dies to produce resin coping patterns.

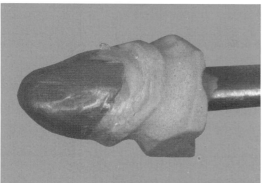

Fig. 11-15b The resin patterns are trimmed with a hot spatula above the die margin. The rough edges are flattened and smoothed with a hot spatula.

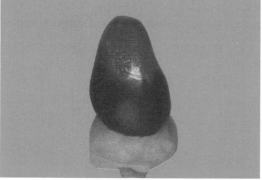

Fig. 11-15c The pattern is extended to the die margin with molten wax. The wax should flow under and over the edges of the plastic thimble.

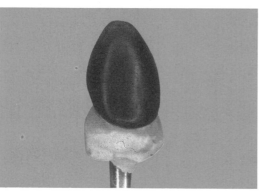

Fig. 11-15d Wax is added over the plastic thimble, building the pattern to ideal coping form.

Fig. 11-16 Wax-dipping technique for a rapid build-up of the coping pattern. The die is dipped into the vat of molten wax to the die margin. Dipping the die twice will build up the wax pattern to approximately one to one and one-half millimeters thick. Waiting a few seconds between dips will facilitate this build-up by allowing the first layer to harden slightly. The margin of the pattern is then refined with a spatula by trimming excess wax or by adding additional wax where needed.

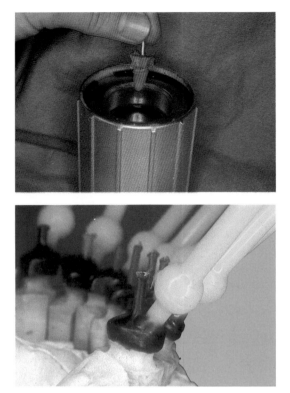

Fig. 11-17 Wax patterns for a short coping sprued with a plastic dowel and ready for investing.

Vacuum-Formed Thimble

Using a thin plastic coping as the pattern is a tremendous aid in forming simple long or medium copings. These thin copings of plastic can be formed with numerous techniques other than by the vacuum-forming process. A vacuum process is preferred by the authors. These patterns are formed in this manner:

1. Select a 0.5 millimeter plastic sheet and insert it into the vacuum machine.
2. Adapt the plastic sheet to the dies under heat and vacuum (Fig. 11-15a).
3. Trim the plastic thimble one millimeter above the die margin and remove the excess sheet (Fig. 11-15b).
4. Flatten the cut surface with a hot spatula.
5. Add molten wax to the plastic coping and to the margin (Fig. 11-15c).

6. Flow additional wax over the plastic coping to increase the thickness, trim the wax margin, sprue, invest, cast and finish the coping (11-15d).

Dipping Technique (Fig. 11-16)

Another simple and rapid technique for coping pattern formation is the wax dipping method. The die is dipped several times into molten wax stored in a special heater. When a sufficient thickness of wax is built up on the die in this manner, the wax is allowed to harden. The wax margin and coping pattern contour is completed and the coping pattern is ready for spruing and investing.

For Short Copings with Dowel Patterns

When the abutments have been prepared for short copings, adding wax to the lubricated die with a hot spatula is preferable. The plastic dowel patterns or metal pins are first inserted into the prepared recesses. The post pattern should extend four to five millimeters beyond the die. Now when wax is added, the exposed post patterns can be used as handles to carefully remove the wax pattern. The added wax is shaped to contour, the margin adjusted and sprued ready for investing (Fig. 11-17).

All coping patterns are invested, cast and polished similar to routine laboratory procedures. These castings can be assembled on the master cast for assembly of attachments, or soldering of all units together.

Chapter 12

Overdenture Framework

A common problem with non-reinforced overdentures is fracturing of the denture base over the abutments (Fig. 12-1). As the alveolar ridge resorbs, the overdenture rests more on the abutments than the soft tissues. The abutments act as wedges, causing splitting or cracking of the overdenture during function. Generally, all overdentures should be reinforced with some form of metal framework. The framework strengthens the overdenture. It may also permit a more compact prosthesis.

Frameworks may vary from a simple retentive meshwork within the denture base to an all-metal saddle, with many variations in between.

The design of an overdenture framework is the responsibility of the dentist (Fig. 12-2). It should be thoroughly outlined on the study cast with complete written instructions submitted to the laboratory technician.

Some of these features must be considered when designing the framework: whether there are long-term or recent extraction edentulous ridges; number of abutment teeth present; where are the abutments located; location of border soft-tissue attachment areas; denture base area to be covered; ridge undercuts; whether the framework will cover the substructure; will the copings be spaced? Where will the copings be spaced? Will the framework be used for taking attachment-retained occlusal records; will the framework be an all-metal base or with a retentive mesh for retaining the denture base?

Overdenture framework design and fabrication is not dramatically different from that for partial dentures. Basically, they may be designed with various forms of major connectors with a metal saddle or some form of retentive mesh for the resin denture base. Special design features as they relate to overdentures will be considered. However, the routine laboratory fabrication procedure, common to most partial denture prostheses, will not be reviewed.

Maxillary Design

Major Connector

The maxillary overdenture framework more commonly involves a horseshoe-shaped major connector (Fig. 12-3). It should be designed somewhat similar to a removable partial denture horseshoe-shaped framework in regards to tissue coverage and anatomical landmarks.

When numerous abutments are retained, the maxillary framework can be fabricated with a very narrow major connector adjacent to the abutments (Fig. 12-4). The acrylic finish line adjacent to and between the abutments can be located next to the lingual surface of the denture teeth. It can be festooned and shaped so that the overdenture appears to be a hybrid fixed-removable bridge. The large edentulous areas should be broader to cover more tissue area for maximum support.

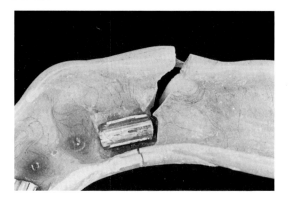

Fig. 12-1 A fractured overdenture without a reinforcing framework. As the alveolar ridge resorbs, stresses are induced in the overdenture near the abutments and it will eventually fracture.

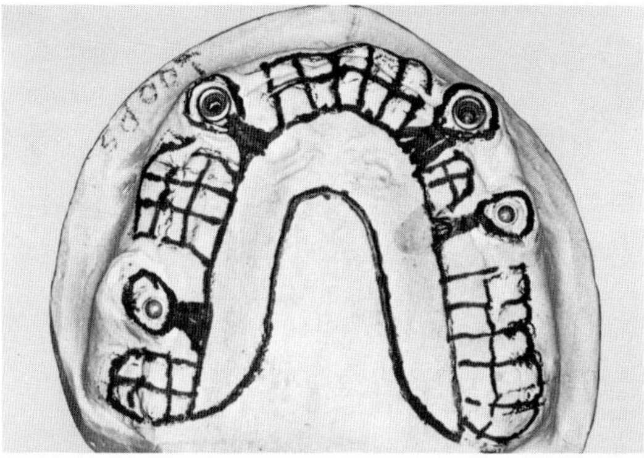

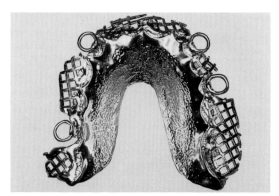

Fig. 12-2 The framework design must be outlined on the cast and sent with a written work authorization to the dental technician. The major connector design shown here is a horseshoe in shape. A metal mesh, or all-metal saddle should be indicated over the alveolar ridge. The framework design may include half or full circle ringlets for solid fixation of the removable attachment component when the framework is to be used for taking occlusal records.

Fig. 12-3 A maxillary framework with a horseshoe-shaped major connector. A metal mesh provides retention for the resin denture base. The lingual finish line is kept close to the lingual surface of the denture teeth to reduce denture bulk.

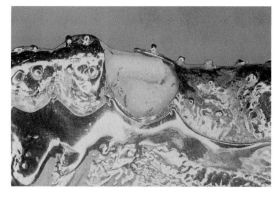

Fig. 12-4 A framework with a very narrow scalloped major connector adjacent to the abutments. The more abutments present, the narrower the major connector can be, somewhat similar to a "quasi" fixed-removable bridge. The edentulous areas should be covered with a wider base for maximum tissue support.

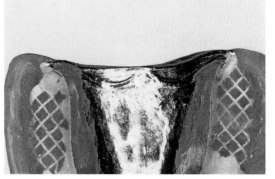

Fig. 12-5 An all-metal full palate framework designed for an overdenture, in long-term extraction situations supported by only a few weak abutments. Such an arrangement provides maximum tissue support. In case of lost abutments the overdenture is easily modified to a complete denture. There is a metal post dam. The removable attachment component can be secured to nearby retentive loops for a root supported and retained occlusal record.

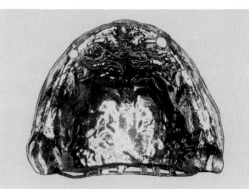

Fig. 12-6 An all-metal palatal framework with retentive provisions provided for a resin post dam. Such post dams are more readily modified than when in metal.

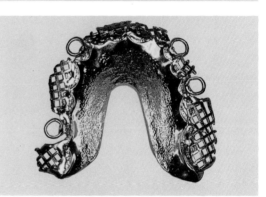

Fig. 12-7 Overdenture framework with mesh frame for retention of the denture base resin. This design is recommended for recent extraction cases when a relining or rebasing procedure may be expected soon.

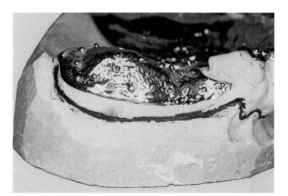

Fig. 12-8 A metal saddle can be used in long-term extraction situations. If the flange periphery is to be the resin denture base, end the framework approximately two millimeters short of the muscle attachment areas. Notice the open area over the cantilevered bar to provide room for the retentive clip. The saddle periphery can end in metal if a muscle-trimmed impression was taken.

When additional rigidity is required, a palatal strap can be added to the horseshoe portion of the major connector. This circular bar form is desirable when only a few abutments support the overdenture.

When only a few questionable abutments are retained, an all-metal palate should be utilized (Fig. 12-5). It should be designed with a metal post dam (Fig. 12-6) or for a resin post dam. Such an overdenture with a full metal palate will provide maximum tissue support and can be easily modified to a complete denture with the loss of the remaining abutments.

A broad-based maxillary major connector should be very thin over most of the palate, particularly when the copings are covered. Strength should be derived with narrow, thick areas supporting broad, thin areas, using the principle of beams. The thicker area near the necks of the denture teeth also add strength to the thinner areas of the major connector.

Minor Connector

In recent extraction situations the framework should be designed with a retentive mesh in the edentulous areas for a resin denture base (Fig. 12-7). In such conditions, the resin denture base is more readily relined or rebased. This meshwork should extend slightly over the crest of the alveolar ridge. If there is inadequate space for denture teeth, end the mesh frame slightly lingual to the crest of the ridge.

In long-term extraction situations, an all-metal denture base can be designed (Fig. 12-8). This metal framework may or may not cover the copings. It should not extend too far anteriorly to present an anterior esthetic problem. Posteriorly, the facial framework should extend several millimeters short of the border muscle attachments if the flange is to end in resin. Or, the posterior periphery can end in metal where esthetics is not a problem. In this latter situation, a muscle-trimmed impression is imperative.

Mandibular Design

Lower frameworks also vary from a simple retentive mesh to an all-metal base or a framework with a metal denture flange. These modifications use most of the principles discussed with maxillary frameworks.

Major Connector

The simplest lower framework uses a retention mesh processed within the acrylic resin denture base to strengthen the overdenture (Fig. 12-9a). This meshwork may be modified to include a lingual bar-like major connector with a definite finish line for the acrylic denture base (Fig. 12-9b). It can be in the form of a very short lingual plate, or modified to a longer lingual plate festooned to receive the denture teeth (Figs. 12-9c and d).

The lower framework may also be fabricated so that the denture flange periphery is partially or completely in metal. The metal flange may extend posteriorly to the bicuspids (Fig. 12-10a); or extend around the retromolar area (Fig. 12-10b). When the lingual bar major connector does extend partly or completely around, it becomes the peripheral edge of the denture flange.

It should be rounded and not knife-like in form, with a definite finish line for the resin denture base.

If the denture flange is to be in metal, the master cast must be produced from a perfectly muscle-trimmed impression. When such an all-metal saddle is fabricated, the authors prefer the entire periphery of the lingual flange end in metal and to extend around to the buccal surface, ending near the bicuspid area facially. The anterior portion should be the resin denture base for esthetics.

General Considerations

Where the framework contacts the tissue, the interfacial surface should represent a

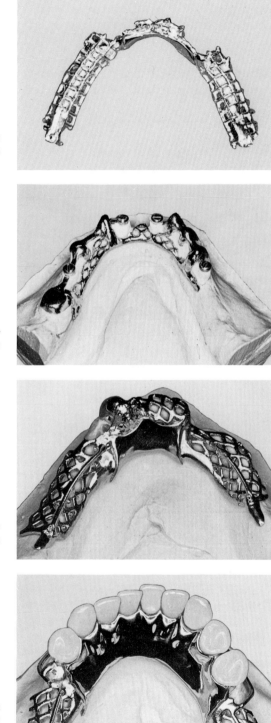

Fig. 12-9 a   A simple lower mesh designed to be processed in the denture base to provide additional strength for the overdenture.

Fig. 12-9 b   A framework with a lingual major connector and a retentive mesh for retention of the resin denture base.

Fig. 12-9 c   A framework with a short lingual plate major connector. Notice the solid metal base covering the lingual half of the copings.

Fig. 12-9 d   A long lingual plate framework. The framework was fabricated to fit directly around the denture teeth, similar to a "tube-tooth" technique.

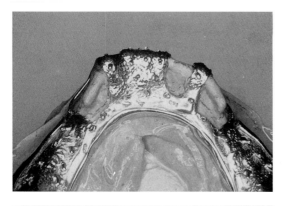

Fig. 12-10a   An all-metal saddle framework with the flange periphery in metal. Openings are provided over the bars to allow room for the retentive shell of the bar attachment.

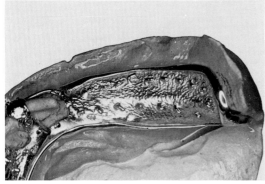

Fig. 12-10b   The metal flange extends over the retromolar pad ending in the bicuspid area for esthetic reasons.

perfect recording of the overdenture-bearing mucosa. The surface should be exceptionally smooth and highly polished (Fig. 12-11).

An all-metal saddle should have provision for mechanically locking the denture resin to the saddle. For this, retentive beads, knobs, or loops may be used (Fig. 12-12). Retentive beads or knobs should be flattened anteriorly so as not to interfere with the set-up of denture teeth.

Often, metal located anteriorly will cause a cosmetic problem when this metal shows through the pink acrylic. Such areas can be covered with a pink opaquing material (Fig. 12-13).

If the overdenture is to be a resilient prosthesis (tissue-tooth supported) and the framework is designed to cover short copings, a one-half millimeter relief should be provided over the coping. Generally in

such a situation alveolar resorption soon eliminates this relief area and the prosthesis soon rests on the copings and soft tissue at the same time. No relief is provided if the overdenture is non-resilient (tooth-tissue supported).

When fabricating a framework that will fit against the copings (for non-resilient cases) a one-half millimeter relief should be provided just over the gingival crest (Fig. 12-14). This space tapers to nothing toward the gingival area of the coping. This will prevent impingement of the denture base on the gingival tissues. However, too much gingival relief here will cause hyperplasia of the soft tissue. This should be avoided.

A tremendous advantage of overdenture techniques is the capability of using the framework as a root-supported and retained occlusal registration base. Such root-retained overdenture frameworks can be

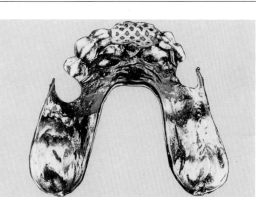

Fig. 12-11 The tissue-contacting areas of the framework must be devoid of all blebs and irregularities and highly polished. This is important to help prevent tissue irritation and promotes overdenture cleanliness.

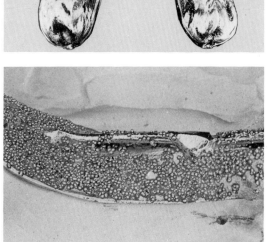

Fig. 12-12 Metal beads or loops provide positive mechanical retention for the denture-base resin. The beads in the anterior region can be flattened slightly to provide additional room for set up of the anterior teeth.

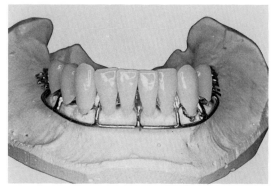

Fig. 12-13 Anterior portions of the framework that may alter the esthetic result by showing through the resin denture flange should be covered with a pink opaquing material.

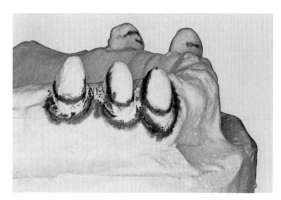

Fig. 12-14 A framework that fits over the coping should be spaced gingivally. Space should be present just over the crest of the gingiva and the undercut portion of the coping; this space should taper to nothing slightly above the coping undercut.

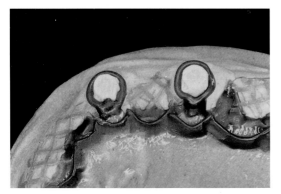

Fig. 12-15 Framework pattern designed with retentive loops for securing attachment for an attachment-retained framework record base.

Fig. 12-15a Pattern with horseshoe-shaped palate and retentive loops for securing the attachments.

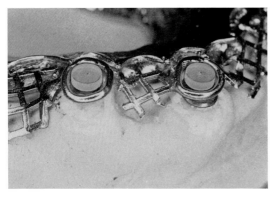

Fig. 12-15b Framework loops fitted around the attachments.

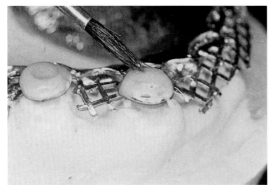

Fig. 12-15c Attachments fixed to the framework with resin.

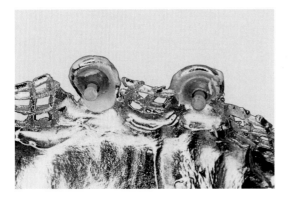

Fig. 12-15d Zest males extending from the framework.

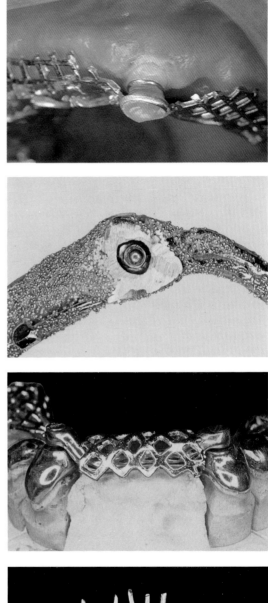

Fig. 12-15e Framework snapped in place with the attachments.

Fig. 12-16 An all-metal saddle framework with holes provided over the stud attachments. The female portion of the stud attachment fits through these holes and is attached to the framework when the framework is used for occlusal records.

Fig. 12-17 The framework meshwork extending over bar attachments must be spaced to allow room for the bar retentive clip.

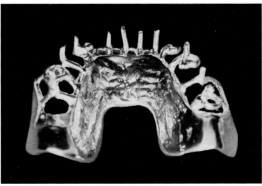

Fig. 12-18 Framework designed for taking functionally generated path records. Such a framework has vertical posts for securing the table for taking functional records in wax. The finished functional casting is secured to these posts.

indispensable feature of specialized occlusal recordings and reconstructive procedures.

If the framework is to be used for taking these abutment-supported and retained occlusal records, the female component of the attachment must be secured to the framework. To lock the female to the framework with acrylic, special mushroom-like knobs or loops must be fabricated on the framework (Figs. 12-15a to e).

When stud attachments are used, provide loops or holes in the metal saddle area over the stud to accommodate the female (Fig. 12-16). When a bar attachment is used, a relief must be fabricated in the framework over the bar to accommodate the retentive clips (Fig. 12-17). In this later case, the framework may have a "window" or be completely open over the bar, particularly if the framework has other areas for retaining the resin denture base (see Figs. 12-4 and 12-10a).

In addition, the framework/attachment assembly can be used for taking other records. For example, it can be used to develop customized anterior guidance and functionally generated path records and then to transform these records into metal to become part of the finished overdenture (see chapter 10). When used in this manner, the framework must be designed with vertical posts extending from the ridge areas of the framework (Fig. 12-18). These techniques will be discussed in more detail later.

Chapter 13

Overdenture Design

As mentioned earlier, the sheer complexity of the oral considerations involved in an overdenture patient can make diagnosis and treatment planning extremely frustrating. Should the overdenture be supported by bare roots? Or should the roots be restored with cast copings? Should the overdenture telescope over the copings? Or is some form of attachment indicated? Which attachment?

In this chapter we outline the indications and disadvantages of each of three basic overdenture designs: bare root, telescopic and attachment fixation overdenture.

Bare Root Overdenture

The overdenture may be placed directly over the crownless, endodontically treated roots, either as an interim step in fabrication or as a final prosthesis (Figs. 13-1a and b).

Indications

1. Roots are used only for conservation of the alveolar ridge and overdenture support (retention and stability are not major concerns).
2. The patient is elderly and in poor health.
3. Time is needed to evaluate questionable teeth.

4. Due to a history of poor oral hygiene, the prognosis for the abutments is questionable.
5. Time is needed to upgrade home care, and evaluate progress before committing the patient to more extensive dental care.
6. Expense is a major consideration.
7. Roots are not involved with caries.
8. Caries index is low.

Disadvantages

1. Provides only stability without retention.
2. The roots are not attached to the rigid prosthesis and therefore are not splinted.
3. The exposed dentine may encourage caries.

Telescopic Overdenture

The roots may be restored with a cast restoration (primary copings), so the prosthesis telescopes over them contacting either directly with the denture acrylic or with metal or porcelain-to-metal (secondary copings, Fig. 13-2).

Indications

1. Roots are retained for conservation of the alveolar ridge.
2. Overdenture support and stability are considerations.

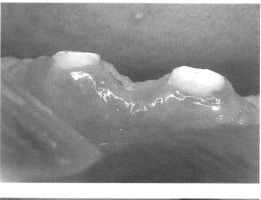

Fig. 13-1a Endodontically treated teeth reduced and shaped to support an overdenture. The coronal opening is closed with silver amalgam. The restoration and root surfaces are smoothed and polished to resist plaque accumulation.

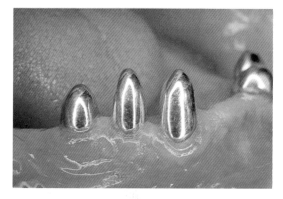

Fig. 13-1b Bare roots shaped like medium copings to provide additional support, stability and some retention to the overdenture. Note the silver amalgam in the canal opening. This is polished later.

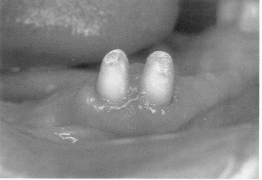

Fig. 13-2 Abutment teeth restored with long primary copings will support an overdenture. The secondary coping that fits over these primary copings will be the denture-base resin.

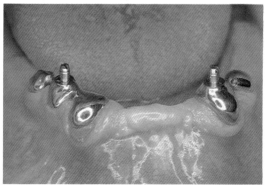

Fig. 13-3 Short copings fitted with special stud attachments will provide retention for the overdenture. The companion component is processed into the denture base. Retentive fixation is accomplished as the overdenture is inserted and when the female snaps over the male stud.

3. Slight retention is desirable.
4. Coping coverage is indicated for caries control.
5. Weak abutments require splinting.
6. The dentist prefers to avoid the complexity of attachments.
7. The patient can afford more extensive overdenture treatment.
8. Good home care habits make long-term prognosis favorable.

Disadvantages

1. Short copings provide no retention.
2. Long or medium copings may provide inadequate retention.
3. Long copings often are too bulky for good esthetics.
4. Since retention of long and medium copings depends on friction alone, it is poorly controlled and troublesome to adjust.
5. Long or medium copings often cannot be used where occlusal space is limited.

Attachment Fixation Overdenture

The overdenture may connect to the copings with studs or other attachment bar-and-rider systems (Fig. 13-3).

Indications

1. Roots are retained for conservation of the alveolar ridge.
2. Overdenture support, stability and retention are all important considerations.
3. Coping coverage is indicated for caries control.
4. Weak abutments require splinting (though some attachments can be utilized without splinting the roots).
5. The dentist desires controlled adjustable retention.
6. Comfort and patient acceptance are major concerns. (An attachment-retain-

ed overdenture feels more like bridgework than a non-attachment overdenture.)
7. The dentist wishes to minimize, or maximize, the amount of denture-bearing mucosa.
8. The dentist desires a more balanced distribution of mastication load between abutments and tissue than is possible with a conventional telescopic overdenture.

Disadvantages

1. More expensive than conventional telescopic overdenture.
2. More difficult to fabricate.
3. More difficult to maintain.
4. Some attachments are bulky and therefore may cause esthetic and occlusal space problems.
5. Patients with limited manual dexterity may have difficulty inserting the prosthesis.

Superiority of Attachment-Fixation Overdenture

The attachment-fixation overdenture is far superior to other types of overdentures or other forms of overlay prostheses. It can more closely approximate the results obtained with fixed bridgework and precision partial denture prosthetics than is possible with telescopic overdentures or complete dentures. The patient is more secure in its use than with a complete denture. Thus, he enjoys increased comfort, function, and a more natural appearance.

Attachment Selection[1]

There is a wide variety of attachments available today for overdenture prostheses and more being developed. Unfortunately,

[1] Attachments available from APM-Sterngold, San Mateo, Calif., or Ultratek, Concord, Calif.

there is no universal system of nomenclature to identify the various attachments. Most attachments have been named after their inventors, e. g., *Gerber, Zest, Dalla Bona* and *Dolder,* to mention just a few. Attachments, however, have certain basic features in common. For example, it may be that extra-coronal attachment, which is located outside the confines of the abutment contour (see Fig. 13-3); or an intra-coronal attachment which is located within the confines of the abutment contour (Figs. 13-4a and b).

For example:

1. Intra-coronal attachments.
    a) Zest
    b) Ginta

2. Extra-coronal attachments.

    a) Studs (*Gerber, Dalla Bona, Rotherman,* etc.).
    b) Bars (*Dolder, Hader,* etc.).
    c) Auxiliary series (Ipsoclip, IC, screws).

Probably the most comprehensive and effective tool for the beginner in attachment identification and attachment selection is the EM attachment selector, developed by Dr. M. C. *Mensor*[1].

Attachment selection need not be a difficult task if selection is based on simple factors common to many attachments. When selecting an attachment, the dentist wishes to use the best attachment in each specific case. There probably is no such thing as "the best attachment," but there may be several attachments that will work equally well. Therefore, attachment selection should not be made by name initially, but should be determined by understanding the basic principles which never change. In fact, attachments customized in the laboratory would probably work just as well as those available from den-

tal manufacturers. However, it is more convenient to purchase these attachments already available.

Whether an extra-coronal or intra-coronal attachment is to be utilized, the dentist must make his selection based upon his knowledge of such factors as a) crown-root ratio desired, b) type of copings, c) vertical space available, d) number of teeth present, e) amount of bone support, f) location of abutments, g) the location of the strongest abutments, and h) whether the overdenture is to be a tooth-supported or a i) tooth-tissue-supported appliance. In addition, such factors as the type of j) opposing dentition is important, for example, whether a complete denture, another overdenture, or natural dentition k) maintenance problems and, of least importance, the l) cost. These selection principles will be considered in detail when discussing the specific attachments.

Finally, to make an intelligent selection, you must also have a thorough understanding of the important features of each specific attachment. It is the authors' recommendation to keep things as simple as possible. For example, select the best attachment of each category and become familiar with and proficient in the use of just these few.

Resilient or Non-Resilient Attachments

Many of the most popular attachments are available in both resilient and non-resilient designs. This is a mechanism for controlling distribution of the forces of mastication uniformly over the denture-bearing mucosa and the supporting abutments. Attachments should be selected on the basis of this action.

1. *A resilient attachment* reduces vertical and lateral forces on the abutments by distributing more of the masticatory load

[1] Bell International, San Mateo, Calif.

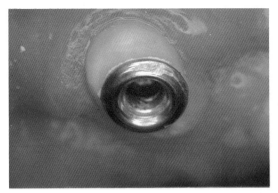

Fig. 13-4 a An intra-coronal attachment, such as the Zest female shown here, is located within the confines of the root.

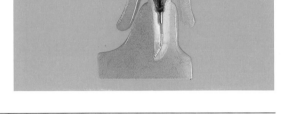

Fig. 13-4 b The male with a spherical head, is processed inside the denture base. When the overdenture is inserted, the male head engages an internal undercut inside the female providing retention and stability for the overdenture.

to the tissues. This is accomplished by fabricating a gap of 0.5-1 millimeter between the overdenture and the metal substructure. When the denture is out of function, it rests entirely on the mucosa. Only during function (after the tissues have compressed 0.5-1 millimeter) are vertical forces transmitted to the substructure and thus to the roots. Resiliency is a special advantage when the denture base fits poorly due to alveolar resorption, faulty fabrication, an inadequately fitted denture base, or errors in cementation of the substructure (the space helps to accommodate the above errors in fit).

Use resilient attachments

a) For a tissue-tooth-supported appliance.

b) With very weak abutments, when maximum tissue support is required.
c) When there are only a few abutments.
d) When functioning opposite natural dentition.
e) When functioning against a non-resilient appliance.
f) When multi-directional action is desired.
g) With minimal denture base.

2. *A non-resilient attachment,* as its name implies, does not permit any vertical movement during function. If the appliance is entirely tooth-supported, the abutments must withstand the entire masticatory load.
   Of course, if the prosthesis rests on the abutments and mucosa at the same time, then the mucosa also supports some of the load during function. An

137

attachment having some rotational movement should be used in such a situation. It compensates for some of the functional loading on the abutments by directing some of these forces to the supporting mucosa.

This maximal loading is less stressful to non-resilient restored abutments when the denture base is broadened and well-adapted to the supporting mucosa.

Use non-resilient attachments

a) When no vertical movement is indicated, but where rotational action may be desirable.
b) With an all-tooth support appliance.
c) With a tooth-tissue-supported appliance.
d) With strong abutments.
e) When functioning against a complete denture.
f) When functioning against a resilient overdenture.
g) With large, well-fitting denture base.
h) Where intra-occlusal space is limited.

Extra-Coronal Attachment Selection

As already mentioned, there are three general types of extra-coronal connectors: stud, bar and auxiliary attachments. Each type has certain characteristics which make it particularly suited to a specific application. First, let's consider the broad selection of an extra-coronal attachment. Your first determination will be to decide which one of the broad category of attachments would be best for the specific conditions.

1. *Bar attachments* (Figs. 13-8a to c)

   a) For splinting abutments.
   b) For retention, stability and support.
   c) Where adequate vertical space is available.

d) Can be used with all coping sizes.
e) Personal preference.

2. *Stud attachments* (Fig. 13-5)

   a) For retention, stability and support.
   b) Where vertical space is limited (depends upon selection of specific stud).
   c) Used generally with short copings.
   d) Can be positioned strategically along a splinted span of abutments.
   e) For maximum tissue support.
   f) Personal preference.

3. *Auxiliary attachments*

   a) Spring-loaded plunger attachment (Fig. 13-6).
      For retention only.
      Generally used to engage the side of long or medium copings.
      May be used for retention with bars.
      Personal preference.
   b) Screws (Fig. 13-7).
      For firm fixation.
      For fixation with another attachment system.
      For specialized conditions.

Bar Attachment Selection

An important feature of the bar attachment is its rigid splinting of the abutments (Fig. 13-8a). However, it requires more space vertically, facially and lingually than a stud attachment. Use the characteristics mentioned earlier, when deciding to use a bar attachment. There are two basic types of bar attachments based on their shape and action provided. For example: 1. Bar Unit and 2. Bar Joint.

1. *Factors to be Considered for Bar Selection*
   Bar Unit – As the name implies, it acts as a fixed unit. This bar has parallel walls providing rigid fixation with frictional reten-

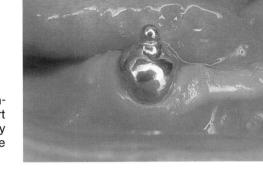

Fig. 13-5 A spherical Dalla Bona stud attachment, is soldered to the diaphragm of a short coping. The male's spherical head is engaged by the retentive clips of the female processed in the denture base.

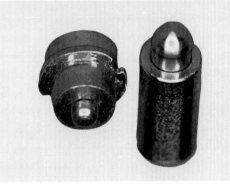

Fig. 13-6 From left to right: Ipsoclip and IC attachments. Plunger attachments generally placed in the secondary coping so that the plunger engages a small depression in the primary coping or a bar. However, the Ipsoclip can be fabricated into the primary coping.

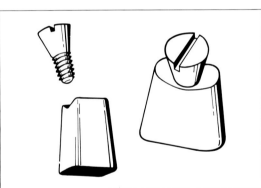

Fig. 13-7 A line drawing of a screw attachment (Hruska). It provides rigid fixation of two separate units that comprise a fixed-removable anchorage system.

tion (Fig. 13-8b). Due to the shape of the bar there will be no rotational or vertical movement of the overlay prosthesis.

This attachment can be used with long, medium or short copings, but only when this appliance is to be tooth supported and no stress-broken action is indicated. It is never used where a bar joint (a movable action) is indicated.

However, a bar joint can be used as a substitute for the bar unit; when the bar joint is not spaced, and when the prosthesis is tooth supported. Thus, selection of a specific bar attachment would depend on its characteristics and the oral conditions.

Bar Joint – It has a curved contour, which permits the prosthesis to rotate around

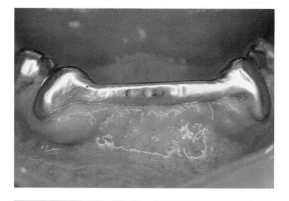

Fig. 13-8a Bar attachments splinting abutments.

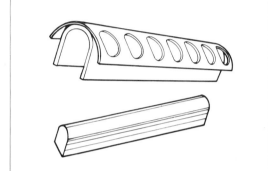

Fig. 13-8b A parallel-walled bar acts as a bar unit. It provides support, stability and retention, but without any provisions for rotational action of the overdenture. The retentive mechanism inside the denture engages the bar providing retention.

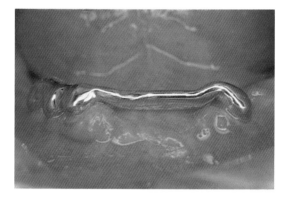

Fig. 13-8c A bar joint is a stress-broken bar anchorage system. Its shape and method of fabrication provides rotational action of the overdenture. In addition, vertical movement of the overdenture may or may not be present depending on how the prosthesis is fabricated.

the bar slightly. This action minimizes the torquing of the bar (and, of course, the roots) during mastication and allows the tissues to assume some of the load (Fig. 13-8c). The bar joint may also feature vertical movement with the prosthesis. Since the typical overdenture case involves weak abutments, the more gentle bar joint is preferred to the rigid modification.

It is a very useful attachment when used under these conditions:

a) Provides vertical and/or rotational action.

b) For retention, support and stability.

c) For splinting abutments.

d) Used with long copings.

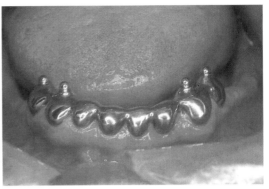

Fig. 13-9a   Multiple spherical Dalla Bona stud attachments on a splinted span of short copings. An important feature of stud attachments is the ability of positioning them strategically along splinted abutments.

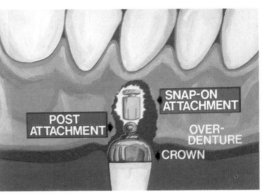

Fig. 13-9b   The female component is processed in the denture base providing retention when the overdenture is inserted. The female retentive lamellae engages the stud ball to produce this retention.

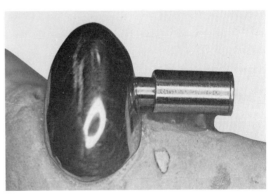

Fig. 13-10   The plunger of the spring-loaded IC attachment engages the round depression in the coping wall. This attachment provides excellent retention for a telescopic overdenture.

e) Used with short copings.

f) Available as resilient.

g) Contraindicated with minimal intra-occlusal space.

2. Listed here are a number of bar attachments that are applicable for removable prosthesis.

a) Dolder bar

b) Hader bar

c) Andrews bar

d) Ceka

e) Octalink

f) C. M. bar

g) M. F. Channels

h) Ackerman bar

i) Customized bars

The specific characteristics of some of these bar attachments will be discussed later in the text.

Stud Attachment Selection

A large variety of stud attachments are available for overdenture use. Most consist of a post-like male secured to the diaphragm of the coping (Fig. 13-9a). The female which engages the male post is processed within the tissue side of the denture. These components engage each other when the overdenture is inserted (Fig. 13-9b). Generally, the retention is obtained by a frictional fit of the female on the male, or a "snap-like" action when the female engages an undercut on the male. Most stud attachments are available as non-resilient or as resilient attachments.

1. *Factors to be Considered for Stud Selection*

   Consider these features when selecting a stud attachment:

   a) Can be used on single copings.
   b) Can be positioned strategically on a coping splint.
   c) May have a much narrower and lower profile. This means that a stud:
   may be used with a short coping for a very favorable crown-root ratio;
   may be used when there is a very limited vertical space;
   permits a highly esthetic overdenture due to its narrow width.
   d) Available in a wide variety of designs from simple to complex.
   e) Available as non-resilient or resilient varieties.
   f) Produces the least bulky overdenture.
   g) For retention, stability and support.

h) Limited in its use on very weak, unsplinted single abutments.

i) Can allow denture movement in several directions.

j) Personal preference.

2. Here are a few examples of some common stud attachments:

   a) Dalla Bona
   b) Gerber
   c) Ceka
   d) Rotherman
   e) Gmur
   f) Huser
   g) Schubiger
   h) Ancrofix

The specific characteristics of some of these stud attachments will be considered in more detail later.

Auxiliary Attachment Selection

Auxiliary attachments are in the category of specialized screws, or spring-loaded plunger types of attachments.
Pressure-button attachments such as the Ipsoclip and IC types have a spring-loaded plunger (see Fig. 13-6). This plunger engages a small depression prepared within the coping or surface of a bar (Fig. 13-10). They can provide auxiliary retention with long or medium copings or bars. They are used only where no rotational movement is programmed into the appliance, although they can be used where vertical resilience is present. Therefore they are often used where abutment teeth are present in more than one plane. The selection of a specific pressure-button attachment would be based upon the characteristics of the particular attachment.

1. *Features of Plunger-type attachments*

   These are some characteristics of the plunger attachment:

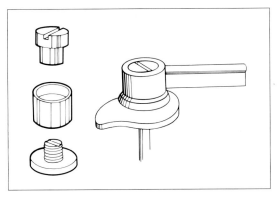

Fig. 13-11a An illustration of the Schubiger screw system. It connects several removable units into a rigid fixed-removable assembly. A screw base is soldered to the coping diaphragm. The removable sleeve portion is connected to a bar.

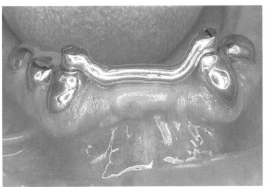

Fig. 13-11b Abutments splinted with a Schubiger-bar assembly. The bar can be removed by unscrewing the sleeves from the Schubiger screw base. As the screw base is common to the Gerber attachment, the Schubiger-bar attachment overdenture can be modified to a Gerber overdenture.

a) Can engage long and medium copings to retain a telescopic overdenture.
b) Can be used to engage bars for retention.
c) Some are self-contained or have replaceable parts.
d) Some can be processed in the acrylic resin denture base, soldered or cast into the secondary coping of an overdenture.
e) May be used to add additional retention to an already existing overlay prosthesis.

2. *Plunger-type attachments*

Listed below are a few of the plunger-type attachments:

a) Ipsoclip
b) Tach-E-Z

c) Presso-matic
d) IC attachment

Of these, the IC attachment is simple in design and use and low in cost, and is frequently used by the authors.

3. *Auxiliary Screw Attachment Selection*

Screws have a rather limited use in overdenture prosthetics, but can become an invaluable adjunct to attachments in special situations. Screw attachments contribute a fixed removable characteristic to an overlay prosthesis and permit easier modification of the prosthesis. Screws may be used for fixation of removable bridgework, for attachment of bars to stud posts and as anchor attachments for individual crowns. Screws would be considered under the following conditions:

1. Fixation with fixed-removable bridgework.
2. For individual crown anchorage.
3. For splinting bars to studded copings on divergent teeth.
4. With a bar prosthesis, where the bar can be removed for easy modification.
5. Personal preference.

4. *Screw Attachments*

The selection of screws is rather limited. Of all the screws, the Schubiger attachment is most widely used in overdenture prosthetics (Figs. 13-11a and b). It is used under most conditions mentioned above, with the exception of single-crown anchorage, and will be considered in more detail later in this text.

The VK-screw system can be used for the fixation of primary copings to roots, or fixation of secondary copings or bars to the supporting abutments.

Chapter 14

Telescopic Overdenture

The telescoped overdenture is an excellent alternative to routine complete dentures. But what exactly is a telescoped or coping overdenture? As the name implies, a telescoped overdenture fits over natural teeth with that portion of the overdenture over the natural teeth fitting like a sleeve. These supporting abutments may simply be endodontically treated teeth reduced slightly, shaped, smoothed, polished and left in this manner to support this denture; or, these roots or teeth may be restored with metal copings. The size of these primary copings, the copings on the teeth, may be medium or long (Fig. 14-1). They may be designed only to provide support, or to provide support and retention.

The secondary copings may be the tissue side of the acrylic denture base, special metal thimbles, or porcelain-to-metal restorations fitted over the primary copings.

Retention is generally obtained through the frictional resistence produced between the semi-parallel walls of the copings and tissue side of the denture base (or secondary coping casting).

Advantages and Disadvantages of Telescopic Overdentures

Advantages

There are numerous advantages with a telescopic overdenture:

1. The retained roots conserve the alveolar ridge.
2. The abutments provide support (and often retention) for a more stable prosthesis.
3. The patient retains some natural proprioception.
4. Because the patient has not "lost all of his teeth," he may emotionally accept the overdenture better than a conventional complete denture.
5. The overdenture permits easy modification should conditions in the mouth change. If abutments fail, it can be converted to a conventional complete denture.
6. Auxiliary retention devices can be added later to a telescopic overdenture.
7. Telescopic overdenture techniques are easy to master. They are a natural transition to attachment fixation overdentures.
8. They are less expensive than attachment fixation overdentures.

Disadvantages

As with all prostheses, there are some disadvantages to the telescopic overdenture:

1. Retention is fixed, and not variable.
2. Retention must be modified frequently.
3. The overdenture is bulky and less esthetic than some attachment overdentures.
4. Though generally less expensive than an attachment overdenture, the telescopic

prosthesis is significantly more expensive than a conventional complete denture.

Overdenture Function

A telescopic overdenture may function in one of three ways: rigid, with masticatory forces directed primarily to the abutments; resilient, with vertical forces directed primarily to the soft tissue; or, stress-broken, with the prosthesis rotating slightly over the abutments.

If there are numerous abutments in two or three planes (or the overdenture will function against either a complete denture or a resilient prosthesis) the rigid design is indicated. Here, the overdenture rests directly on the abutments in the passive position. This means that during mastication, forces will be transferred to the mucosa only to the degree that the abutments are compressed in their sockets.

Because the typical overdenture candidate has so few teeth and because the teeth are usually so unstable, most telescopic overdentures are either resilient or stress-broken to reduce forces on the abutments. When only a few teeth remain, and they are located in several planes, the overdenture should be resilient. The resilient design is identical to the rigid design with one exception. A 0.5-1.0 mm spacer foil is placed over each coping before the prosthesis is fabricated. This leaves a gap between overdenture and coping, so that the abutment will start bearing masticatory load only after the mucosa has been compressed (as the alveolar ridge resorbs, the overdenture may come to rest directly on the abutment, and hence, become a rigid overdenture).

When the few remaining abutments are located in a single plane, the overdenture should be stress-broken rather than resilient. The stress-breaking rotation is created by spacing the facial and lingual surfaces of the primary and secondary copings.

During mastication the occlusal of the primary coping acts as a fulcrum around which the prosthesis rotates, so the posterior mucosa will assume a significant portion of the load. No allowance for vertical movement should be made if rotational action is provided.

Coping Design

No telescopic overdenture treatment is possible without a thorough understanding of the various coping designs and their function. Since this subject has been extensively covered earlier, please refer to the chapter on "Coping Design" for review.

A Telescopic Overdenture Treatment

Procedure

This patient was a fifty-five-year-old female with advanced periodontal disease and extensive breakdown of the natural dentition (Fig. 14-2). The teeth were devitalized and restored with short and long copings to support an overdenture in the following manner:

1. Examination, diagnosis and treatment plan.
2. Study casts for fabrication of interim overdentures.
3. Prophylaxis, soft tissue curettage and home care instructions.
4. Reduction of the abutment teeth, six to eight millimeters for long copings; and four to six millimeters for medium copings. Section through the clinical crowns with a high-speed fissure bur. First you may cut partially through the facial surface and next partially through the lingual surface. The sectioned crown can then be gently snapped off with a small chisel. Reduce each tooth similarly (Fig. 14-3a).

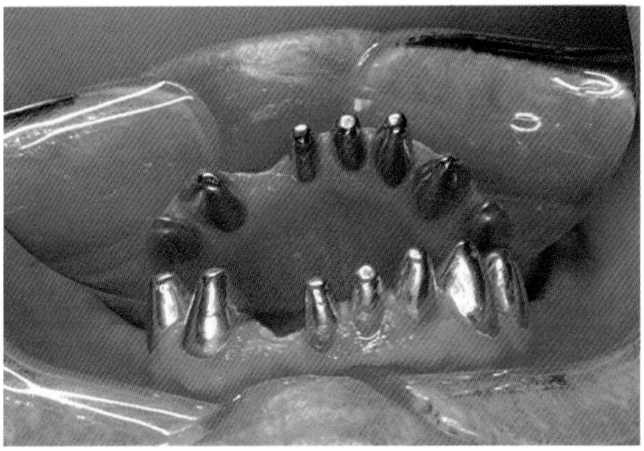

Fig. 14-1 Abutment teeth restored with copings will support a telescopic overdenture. The copings, medium to long, are designed for support and retention.

Fig. 14-2 A patient with signs of extreme dental neglect, particularly with advanced periodontal disease associated with extensive bone loss. A poor candidate for routine restorative procedures, but excellent for a telescopic overdenture.

Fig. 14-3a Abutments are sectioned with a fissure bur and high-speed handpiece. This initial reduction is determined by the proposed coping length. Keep in mind that this occlusal level may require reduction after periodontal surgery and healing and maturation of the periodontium. The abutments will be longer after this healing.

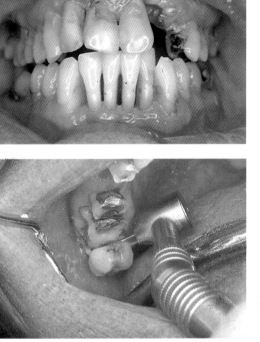

Fig. 14-3b The reduced abutment teeth were managed with preliminary endodontic therapy. A cotton pledget moistened with medicament was sealed into the canal enlargement with a temporary stopping.

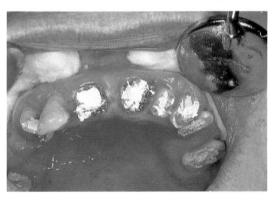

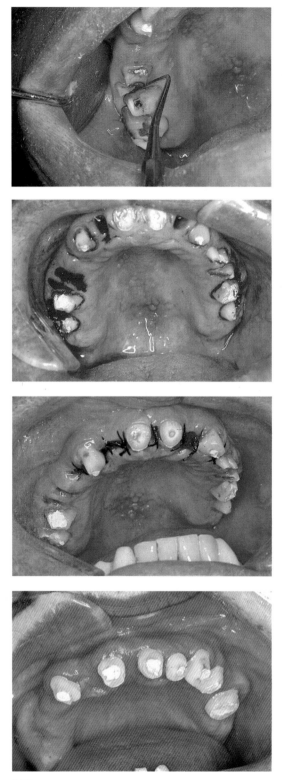

Fig. 14-3c   Abutments are rough-prepared. The hopeless roots of multiple-rooted teeth are sectioned and removed as the clinical crowns are prepared. The roughly prepared roots help to stabilize and retain the interim overdenture.

Fig. 14-3d   The teeth and roots of multiple-rooted teeth, with a hopeless prognosis for overdentures, were removed.

Fig. 14-3e   Periodontal surgery was performed on the remaining abutments. An interim overdenture is a valuable aid in treatment, replacing the missing teeth and clinical crowns, as well as acting as a periodontal bandage.

Fig. 14-3f   Final preparation of the abutments is completed after healing and maturation of the gingival tissues. The centrals were prepared for short copings. All other teeth were prepared for medium or long copings.

5. For those teeth sectioned through the vital pulps, endodontics is mandatory. With a number 4 bur, enlarge the occlusal opening of the canal to a depth of two to three millimeters. This will provide space for the cotton pledget moistened with medicament and temporary stopping.

6. You may wish to initiate or complete the endodontics at this time. In this case, endodontic therapy was only partially completed and a medicament sealed into each canal (Fig. 14-3b).

7. The abutments were partially prepared with an appropriate diamond bur – similar to routine crown and bridge preparations (Fig. 14-3c).

8. Remove all teeth scheduled for extraction (Fig. 14-3d).

9. Since periodontal therapy was not completed earlier, it was performed at this time. It is important to conserve as much bone as possible during periodontal surgery, since most such retained teeth have minimal bone support (Fig. 14-3e).

10. The patient was provided with a previously constructed interim overdenture relined to the surgical site, as in the technique discussed earlier in the text. This interim denture was worn for three months, until the tissues had healed and matured.

11. After healing, the preparations were modified to receive medium or long copings. Short copings are to be placed on the two centrals. The other abutment teeth were prepared to receive long or medium copings (Fig. 14-3f). The overall preparation for the longer copings were tapering with a rounded occlusal or incisal. A chamfer, or small shoulder with a beveled marginal preparation, is prepared. This marginal preparation is determined primarily by the type of primary and secondary coping. If the secondary coping was a crown rather than a hollowed denture tooth, then the shoulder preparation must be more

substantial. The final preparation of the teeth should result in a tapered cone-shaped abutment rather than a rounded occlusal or incisal. This preparation should extend to the gingival sulcus as for a full crown preparation. Sufficient tooth structure was removed facially to make room for the coping and set-up of the anterior teeth, thus ensuring a more esthetic result. The short anterior abutments were prepared for dowel post retention.

12. An impression was taken of the prepared abutment teeth for coping fabrication only.

13. The impression was poured to produce a master cast with removable dies for fabrication of the copings (Fig. 14-4). The long copings were designed for retention and stability; the two short copings were designed for support and stability only.

14. The copings were tested for fit on the abutments and then cemented in place (Fig. 14-5).

15. Now an impression was taken of the denture bearing mucosa and copings to produce a master-cast for fabrication of the overdenture.
This master impression is a very important step, as the sawing, cutting, and trimming of dies invariably destroys the tissue areas of the original cast. These areas cannot be accurately replaced with plaster. Therefore it is always recommended that these primary copings be first cemented on the abutments, and then a master impression taken for fabrication of the overdenture, as discussed above.

16. The master casts are mounted on an appropriate articulator with accurate occlusal records (Fig. 14-6).

17. All coping undercuts are blocked out with plaster (Fig. 14-7).

18. A metal framework with a horseshoe-like major connector was fabricated on a refractory model made from the master

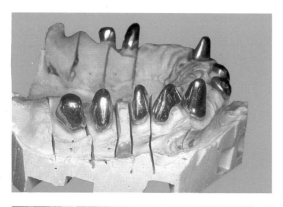

Fig. 14-4   Completed copings on a master cast ready for cementation on the abutments. The overdenture should not be fabricated on this cast. The sawing and trimming of dies destroys their usefulness for this purpose. It is impossible to modify or replace with plaster the stone material destroyed by cutting and trimming of these dies.

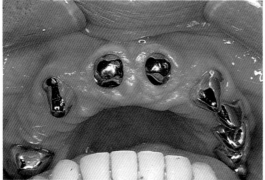

Fig. 14-5   Copings cemented on the prepared abutments. A more accurate master cast is produced when an impression is taken with the castings cemented in place. It is this master cast that should be used for fabrication of the overdenture. This simple procedure eliminates any errors in the fit and cementation of the copings; it also eliminates the problem caused by the sawing and trimming of the dies.

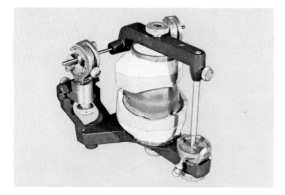

Fig. 14-6   Master casts articulated on an appropriate articulator with accurate intra-occlusal records. Simple custom trays with occlusal rims may be used to obtain these records. A root-retained framework used as the recording device will produce more accurate records.

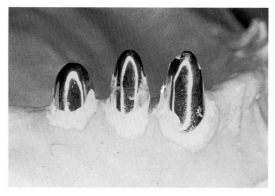

Fig. 14-7   All coping undercuts are blocked out with plaster. This prevents denture-base resin from being processed into the undercut areas thus preventing insertion of the overdenture. When such undercuts are poorly blocked out often it is difficult to determine the area of interference when the overdenture is inserted. If the undercuts are over-blocked out, space will be present into which soft tissue will proliferate.

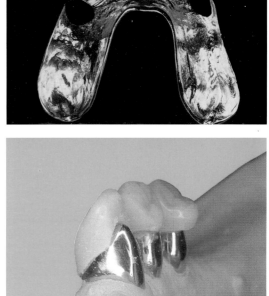

Fig. 14-8   A framework pattern for reinforcing the overdenture. The framework consists of a horse-shoe-shaped major connector and a retentive mesh for the resin denture base.

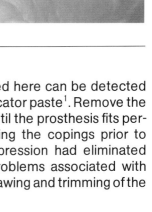

Fig. 14-9   Resin denture teeth "hollow" ground to fit in close contact with the copings. This provides space for maximum esthetics when inadequate room exists for the anterior teeth produces unnatural results. A number 8 bur is recommended to adjust these teeth to fit over the copings, using a large stone to perform this function ends in a "mutilated" result.

cast (Fig. 14-8). Review the Chapter 12, "Framework Design."

19. The properly designed and fabricated maxillary framework was positioned on the cast in preparation for the articulation of the denture teeth.

20. The denture teeth were set up and checked with the patient for occlusion and esthetics. Resin denture teeth were hollow-ground to fit closely to the copings for maximum esthetics (Fig. 14-9).

21. The denture set-up was waxed, festooned, flasked, packed and finished similar to routine full denture fabricating techniques (Fig. 14-10).

22. The telescopic overdenture was inserted in place over the previously cemented copings. If the overdenture does not fit perfectly for some reason, be suspicious that the coping undercuts were not adequately blocked out with plaster.

Resin processed here can be detected with a spot indicator paste[1]. Remove the excess resin until the prosthesis fits perfectly. Cementing the copings prior to the master impression had eliminated overdenture problems associated with coping fit and sawing and trimming of the dies.

As discussed earlier in the text, the resin denture base fitted over the primary copings are actually the secondary copings (Fig. 14-11). A resin secondary coping of a telescoped overdenture does have some advantages over a metal secondary coping – particularly where no auxiliary retentive means are used. It is easier to adjust the retention by adding auto-polymerizing resin to the previously relieved secondary coping spaces and

[1] The J. M. Ney Co., Bloomfield, Ct.

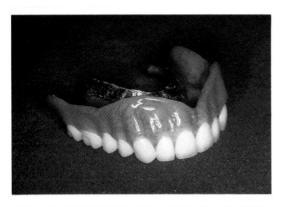

Fig. 14-10 Completed overdenture ready for insertion over the cemented copings.

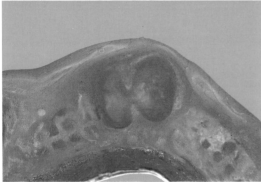

Fig. 14-11 The hollow spaces in the denture base act as secondary copings that fit over cemented primary copings. Retention is provided by the frictional fit of the primary and secondary copings (the hollow denture space). Retention is adjusted by relining the secondary coping with tissue-colored auto-polymerizing resin.

relining the coping spaces directly in the mouth. It is done in this manner: 1. relieve the secondary coping spaces to provide room for the relining resin; 2. place a small amount of mixed tissue-colored resin into the spaces; 3. when the mix becomes slightly doughy, repeatedly insert and remove the prosthesis until the resin hardens; 4. remove all excess flash of resin material.

Relining and/or Rebasing

As the alveolar ridges resorb, the overdenture will begin to rock and direct damaging lateral stresses to the abutment teeth. Now the prosthesis must be adjusted for a better fit by relining or rebasing. This is a simple procedure and performed similar to any complete denture relining or rebasing procedure: 1. hollow out the secondary resin coping to provide adequate room for the impression material; 2. paint an adhesive material on the denture base; 3. load the tissue area of the overdenture with an elastic impression material; 4. insert the overdenture in position and have the patient close gently into occlusion as you muscle-trim; 5. now the overdenture is relined or rebased similar to any complete denture technique and ready for use.

Chapter 15

The Zest Anchor Attachment

As already mentioned, overdentures supported by plain root stubs are far superior to the full denture resting on the edentulous ridges. But these simple root-supported overdentures can be made even more effective by incorporating an intracoronal root attachment such as the Zest anchor.

The Attachment

The Zest anchor is an ideal attachment for use with an overlay prostheses to provide retention and support. The fact that this particular attachment can be used with or without copings makes it an ideal attachment when economy or an intermediate treatment plan is a consideration.

This attachment system has numerous components. As shown in the illustration (Fig. 15-1), from right to left: female, white male post with spacer, blue transfer post with spacer, support cap, red substitute female, ceramic rod with female, sizing drill and number forty-two drill.

Attachment Function

Briefly, the female is cemented within a special recess prepared inside the occlusal portion of a non-vital root with a special sizing bur (Fig. 15-2). The nylon male, which provides retention, is processed within the tissue side of the overdenture (Fig. 15-3). Positive retention and support are accomplished when the terminal ball portion of the male engages the internal undercut of the female when the denture is inserted (Fig. 15-4).

Zest Anchor Components (Fig. 15-1)

Listed below are various Zest components.

1. Diamond sizing bur. This special diamond bur is used to prepare a recess in the root to receive the female portion of the Zest anchor. It is available for a standard female and mini-female. It is also available to fit either a latch-type or a friction-grip handpiece.
2. Female. This portion of the attachment, which is cemented in the prepared root, is available in standard size, for large roots and in a mini-size for smaller roots.
3. White nylon male. This male post is processed in the tissue side of the denture base. It engages the female undercut when the overdenture is inserted.
4. Male centering sleeve. The male centering sleeve fits over the male post and aids in accurately positioning the male inside the female during fabrication for effective retention.
5. Support cap. The support cap permits the dentist to fit a root with a female, yet not activate it for retention. Since it has no terminal ball, it only provides vertical and lateral support to the denture overlay.
6. Blue transfer male. This simulated male with its centering sleeve, is used

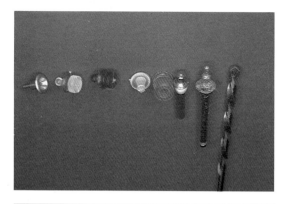

Fig. 15-1 Components of the Zest anchorage system (from left to right): female, white male post with spacer, blue transfer post with spacer, support cap, red substitute female, ceramic rod with female, sizing drill and number forty-two drill.

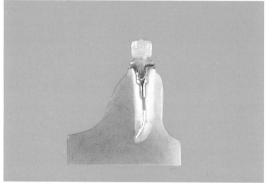

Fig. 15-2 A female component cemented into a previously prepared recess. An internal undercut inside the female will be engaged by the ball-like male provides the overdenture retention. Notice how the flat portion of the female fits flush on the root surface like an inlay. The terminal narrow rod-like extension of the female provides additional retention in the root.

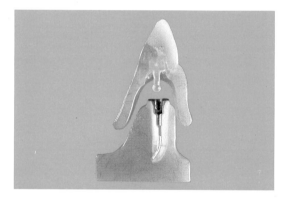

Fig. 15-3 The nylon male with its terminal ball-like knob engages the internal undercut of the female. The male will be retained within the denture base through its round disc-like base.

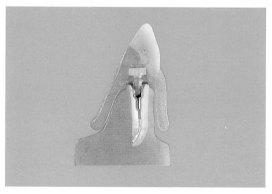

Fig. 15-4 Cross section view showing the overdenture in place with the male engaging the female undercut. The wide flare of the female provides space for rotational movement of the male. Note the small space under the male post. This space accommodates a small degree of vertical movement. Now when the abutments are spaced the overdenture is capable of approximately 0.5 mm vertical translation.

during relining procedures, or during original fabrication when using the indirect technique for positioning the white male posts inside the denture. Its diameter is smaller than that of an actual male (the white male post). Therefore it is more easily removed with the master impression. The transfer male is discarded after denture fabrication.

7. Red substitute female. Used with the blue transfer males for the techniques described above.

8. Male spacer. Used to create a space within the denture base, so the regular male post can be picked up directly in the mouth using self-curing resin.

9. Ceramic rod with female attachment. This assembly is used to place a metal female into the wax coping pattern to produce a gold casting with a metal female.

10. Number forty-two drill. Used to make a hole in the middle of the root on the master cast to receive a male spacer. This technique is used when the male is to be positioned directly in the denture in the mouth.

Zest Overdenture Procedure

Like all overdenture treatments, a Zest anchor overdenture begins with a thorough oral examination, diagnosis and a careful treatment plan. This examination should include casts mounted on an appropriate articulator with accurate intra-occlusal records. A periodontal evaluation using a periodontal probe and radiographs will help determine which roots are to be retained. Roots of teeth having the most bone support and in the most strategic location should receive the attachments for retention. Roots of teeth not adequately supported by bone, or in an undesirable location, need not be used for retention – but only for support to conserve the alveolar ridge.

Whenever possible, periodontal surgery should be completed several months prior to the operative appointment. Of course, the reduction of the teeth makes endodontics mandatory. Endodontics must be completed prior to insertion of the female attachment.

Basic Techniques

There are two basic techniques for managing the patient with a Zest anchored overdenture.

The indirect approach involves the prior positioning of the females into endodontically treated teeth. Then transfer males are placed into the females and a master impression is taken of the denture-bearing area and the roots with the females fitted with transfer males. The transfer males are withdrawn with the impression, and females snapped over the posts so that a master cast is produced with substitute females accurately positioned on the cast. The overlay prosthesis is fabricated on the casts in such a way that the males become accurately fabricated in the denture base.

The direct approach involves the prior fabrication of the overlay prosthesis without males. After the overlay prosthesis is delivered to the dentist, the endodontically treated teeth are fitted with the females. The males are then locked into special recesses within the denture directly in the mouth with self-curing resin.

The following patient treatment involves a seventy-one year old female to be fitted with a Zest retained maxillary overdenture supported by four abutments.

Indirect Procedure

Here is a brief description of the steps in the indirect procedure.

1. Examination, diagnosis, treatment plan.
2. Periodontal therapy and endodontics.
3. Prepare the roots.
4. Insert females into roots.

5. Place transfer males into cemented females.
6. Take master impression for the overlay prosthesis with the withdrawn transfer males in position.
7. Place red substitute females or, preferably, regular females over the males in the impression.
8. Pour impression to produce a cast with transfer females locked in position.
9. Take occlusal registration.
10. Set up and articulate teeth.
11. Place white males on the cast inside the females.
12. Process overlay prosthesis with males in place.

Root Preparation and Seating of Females

1. For this treatment all peridontal therapy and extractions were completed several months prior to the initial operative appointment.
2. Use a high-speed handpiece with a carbide fissure bur to reduce the teeth to approximately 3-4 mm above the gingival tissues initially (Fig. 15-5).
3. If endodontics has not been previously completed, it may be accomplished at this time. Such treatment is greatly simplified by the prior removal of the crown and reduction of the root. With improved access to the canal of the tooth, the canal can be mechanically manipulated with a reduction gear contra-angle and appropriate drills, a special contra-angle with latch-type reamers, or with hand instrumentation. Only the apical portion of the root is filled to allow adequate room for the post of the female.
4. Each root surface is now reduced with a diamond bur in the same plane slightly above the gingiva (Fig. 15-6). This adjustment cut is made at right angles to the path of insertion of the overdenture (in relation to soft tissue undercuts and the pulp canal of

each tooth). When making this cut, or reduction, stop when 0.5 to 1.0 millimeter from the gingiva (at its nearest point). This produces the most favorable crown-root ratio, with little danger of the female being below the gingival crest. Remember, the root surface must be high enough to permit a round periphery. The cut and contoured surface should not be submerged below the gingiva. Otherwise, the gingiva will proliferate over the abutments.

5. To prepare a recess into the canal drill a six millimeter pilot hole into the canal with a number two round bur (Fig. 15-7). Drill these pilot holes parallel to each other and to the path of insertion. When making the pilot holes where the females are not to follow the root canal, due to differences in the path of insertion and because of the soft tissues and bone undercuts, care should be exercised so as not to perforate the root wall. When preparing recesses in multiple-rooted teeth, do not perforate the pulpal floor.
6. Next, enlarge the occlusal three to four millimeters of the pilot hole with a fissure or number six round bur to a size slightly smaller than the main body of the female (Fig. 15-8). This eliminates excess drilling with the sizing bur.
7. Prepare the female recess with the special diamond sizing bur (Fig. 15-9). It is best to use a reduction gear contra-angle[1] at a slow speed to avoid excessive movement that might over-size the recess, or even break the post portion of the drill. If the opening is inadvertently made too large so the female does not fit snugly, fill the recess with amalgam or a composite filling material and re-prepare. If the canal cannot be followed, remove both the post portion of the drill and the female, or, use the mini-drill and mini-female. The hole should be drilled so that a very, very slight recess is also

[1] Whaledent International, New York, N.Y.

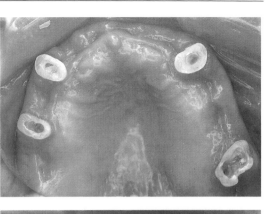

Fig. 15-5 Abutment teeth intially reduced, with a carbide fissure bur, to three to four millimeters above the gingiva. The clinical crowns are cut in the same plane and at right angles to the path of insertion. This path of insertion is determined by ridge undercuts and long axis of the abutments.

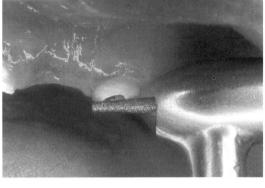

Fig. 15-6 Final preparation as the root surfaces are reduced, with a diamond bur, to approximately one millimeter above the nearest area of the gingiva. Terminating the root preparation here prevents the root surface from being below the crest of the gingiva.

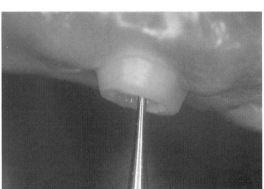

Fig. 15-7 Pilot holes drilled into each root, with a number two bur, to a depth of six to eight millimeters. This hole aids the penetration of the post portion of the sizing bur.

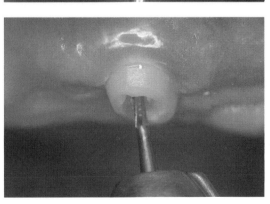

Fig. 15-8 The occlusal three to four millimeters of the canal are enlarged with a fissure bur. The diameter of this opening must be smaller than the diameter of the sizing bur. Enlarging the canal reduces drilling with the diamond sizing bur.

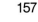

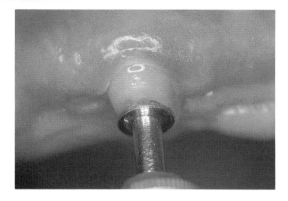

Fig. 15-9 Female recess prepared with the diamond sizing bur. The drill is held parallel to the overdenture's determined path of insertion. When the long axis of the root is divergent from the path of insertion, exercise care so as not to penetrate the side of the root. A slight seat to receive the female flange is also cut into the root surface. The bur is held steady so as not to enlarge the recess.

created on the occlusal root surface with the disc portion of the drill. The female will fit into this recess like an inlay.

8. The females are now ready to be cemented into the roots. Mix the crown and bridge cement to the proper consistency for cementing an inlay. Introduce cement deep into the recess with a lentulo spiral drill[1]. Next, insert a male attachment into the female with the centering sleeve in position (Fig. 15-10a). Add cement to the female, and using the inserted male as a handle, insert the female into the recess. Keep firm pressure on the male until initial set of the cement (Fig. 15-10b).

9. After final set of the cement, remove the male post and all excess cement.

10. The root surface is now ready for final preparation and finishing. With a fine diamond bur, remove all sharp corners at the root periphery. Contour, shape and drill toward the gingival margin, but end this contour and root margin approximately 0.5 millimeter above the gingiva (Fig. 15-11). Finally, polish the root surface with appropriate discs and rubber wheels.

Indirect Procedure for Processing Males into the Denture

1. After females have been cemented into

the roots, the blue transfer posts, with their centering sleeves, are now inserted into the females in each root. These male posts have slightly less retention than that of the white males, and will be withdrawn easily with the impression (Fig. 15-12).

2. On a previously fabricated study cast, construct a custom tray for a master impression. Drill holes through the tray over the area of the male posts. These holes minimize possible distortion or dislodgement of the male transfer posts.

3. Since the teeth are reduced to the gingival crest, the arch can be treated as if it were edentulous. Therefore, the tray is muscle-trimmed with molding compound to produce an accurate record of the peripheral soft tissue attachments. A master impression may be taken with a zinc oxide impression paste; or even rubber-base impression material. Record the denture-bearing ridge area and the roots with their females. The transfer posts are then withdrawn within the impression material. This impression can be made with the impression material of your choice.

4. When the impression is removed, you will notice the ends of the male posts extending out of the impression material (Fig. 15-13). Place spare females or the red substitute females over the ends of these transfer males. These females

[1] Medidenta, Woodside, N.Y.

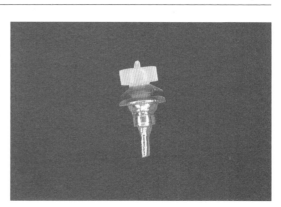

Fig. 15-10a   Before cementing the female into the prepared recess, a male post is first inserted into the female to act as a handle facilitating the cementation process.

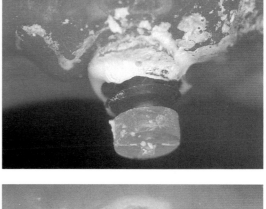

Fig. 15-10b   The female is cemented in the root recess. After the cement sets, the male post and excess cement are removed.

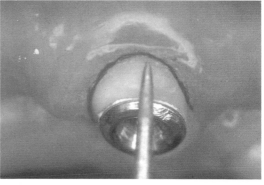

Fig. 15-11   Root surfaces are contoured with a fine grit bur. Sharp corners of the roots are rounded off toward the gingiva. The cut surface is polished with a fine rubber point and rubber cups with tin oxide abrasive.

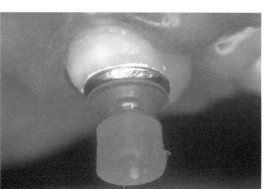

Fig. 15-12   Blue transfer males with centering sleeve positioned in the females. These male posts are smaller in diameter than the white posts, so are easier to remove with an impression. The centering sleeve is pressed snugly into the females. The centering sleeve stabilizes the males with its ball engaging the female undercut.

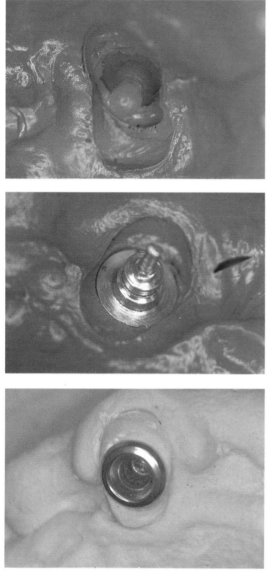

Fig. 15-13 The blue transfer male is withdrawn with the overdenture impression. Note the end of the male extruding from the impression. The hub of the male is securely anchored in the impression material. Impression material injected under the hub prior to taking the impression will assure firm retention of the male.

Fig. 15-14 A metal female is snapped in position over the blue male prior to pouring the impression with model stone. A definite snap should be felt as the female is inserted. A red substitute female may be used instead of the metal female for this purpose.

Fig. 15-15a The females placed on the blue transfer males are now an integral part of the master cast and in the same relationship as in the mouth.

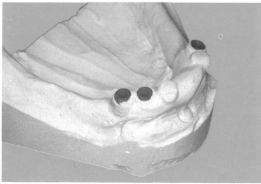

Fig. 15-15b Regular metal females lead to fewer problems than the plastic substitute females shown here. There is a tendency for thin layers of stone to flake off the red substitute females, thus destroying the accuracy of the master cast.

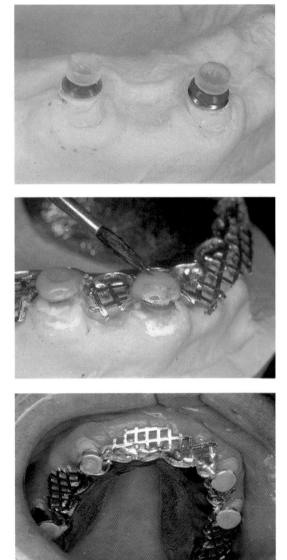

Fig. 15-16a   Zest male inserted in a substitute female on the master cast.

Fig. 15-16b   Male posts locked to the metal framework with auto-polymerizing resin.

Fig. 15-16c   This metal framework, when fitted with an occlusal wax rim, now becomes the occlusal registration tray. A more stable relationship is produced as the males engage the undercuts of the females.

must be snapped firmly over the posts, but with care so as not to dislodge the males (Fig. 15-14).

5. Pour the cast using the impression, with the transfer females locked securely in place. The transfer females now become an integral part of the master cast (representing the females in the patient's mouth, Figs. 15-15a and b).

6. The master cast for the fabrication of the overdenture is now completed.

7. This master cast is used to fabricate a occlusal tray with wax rims for occlusal registration. This occlusal tray may be a shellac tray, a tray made of self-curing resin, or even the metal framework used as part of the final prosthesis.

8. For added retention and stability when

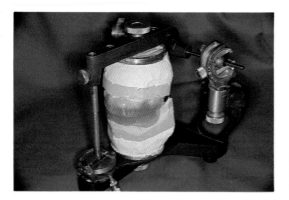

Fig. 15-17 a Casts articulated with the root-retained occlusal record for set-up of the denture teeth.

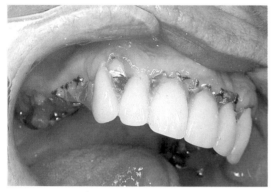

Fig. 15-17 b The set-up can be snapped directly in the mouth to check for accuracy of the occlusal records, as well as for the patient's acceptance of esthetics.

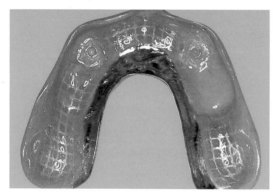

Fig. 15-18 Fabricated Zest-retained overdenture with the end of the male post extending from the denture base. The male spacer and all resin flash is removed from around the post.

you take occlusal records, the tray may be fitted with the white Zest males. To do this, place a hole in the tray over each transfer female to receive the white male posts. Lock the male to the tray or metal framework, with a hard wax or self-curing resin (Figs. 15-16b and c). Use of the white males during occlusal registration also aids in the set-up of the denture teeth.

9. Occlusal records are now taken with the technique of your choice.
10. The occlusal records are used to articulate the casts on an appropriate articulator.
11. Before set-up of the denture teeth, in-

sert the white male firmly into each female. Push down each centering sleeve to accurately position each male. This makes the ball of the male firmly engage the female undercut for maximum retention.

12. Block out all undercuts around the roots with plaster.
13. Set up the denture teeth. The denture set-up is then checked in the mouth for occlusion and any esthetic modification (Figs. 15-17a and b).
14. Wax, festoon, flask, pack and finish as you would any conventional complete denture.
15. Remove the centering sleeve and excess flash from around each male post. The overdenture is now ready for insertion (Fig. 15-18).

Direct Technique

In the direct technique, the overdenture is first fabricated without the Zest males. The females are placed into the abutments, the males snapped into the females, and then locked directly into the overdenture in the mouth. The recess inside the overdenture to receive the males either can be prepared chairside by the dentist, or processed into the overdenture using special male spacers. The following procedure describes the direct technique using male spacers to prepare a recess inside the overdenture to receive the male directly in the mouth.

1. Using the procedure of your choice, take a master impression of the denture-bearing ridge areas and existing dentition. The resulting cast will be treated similar to that for an immediate denture insertion.
2. Fabricate custom trays for recording the occlusal registration. Mount the casts on an appropriate articulator.
3. Trim the teeth on the cast to simulate the reduced abutments. Remove the teeth on the cast that are to be extracted later (Fig. 15-19a).

4. Using a number forty-two drill in a straight handpiece, prepare a hole in the cast of each root that will be fitted with a Zest female. Following the long axis of each tooth, drill the holes parallel to the path of insertion (Fig. 15-19b).
5. Insert the special red male spacers into these holes (Fig. 15-19c). The spacers assist in the set-up of the teeth by providing adequate room for the nylon male. If the holes are drilled correctly, the male spacers should be in correct position over each root. The spacers will be removed after the overdenture is processed, leaving a recess in the tissue side of the denture to accommodate the hub of the white male. You may make adjustments to these recesses, or to the nylon male, if necessary.
6. Set up the denture teeth, articulate, wax, and festoon as you would a conventional complete denture (Fig. 15-19d).
7. The denture is half-flasked, full-flasked, processed and polished with the spacer in place.
8. Remove the male spacers leaving recesses within the overdenture base to receive the male posts (Fig. 15-19e). The overdenture is now delivered to the dentist for insertion.
9. Now the teeth must be prepared to receive the Zest females. The endodontically treated teeth are prepared to receive the females as described earlier. The females are cemented and the denture is ready for insertion and positioning of the male posts.
10. Any teeth to be removed should be extracted at this time.
11. Next, test the fit of the overdenture to be certain that it sits passively on the tissues when it is in position. If any rocking is present, remove any denture material that may be impinging upon the prepared roots or the females.
12. Place a small amount of vaseline into the females before inserting the males. This prevents self-curing resin from getting

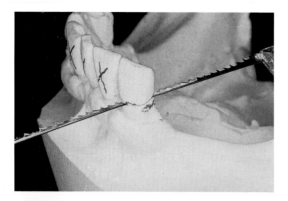

Fig. 15-19a   Abutments on the cast, to receive the females, are trimmed to approximately the same height as that in the mouth. The teeth to be extracted are removed from the cast.

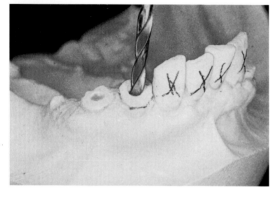

Fig. 15-19b   A hole is drilled into the model of each tooth with a number forty-two drill. The hole is drilled parallel to the path of insertion.

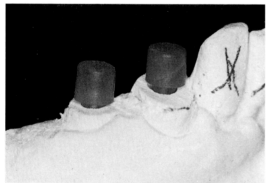

Fig. 15-19c   A red male spacer is inserted into the drilled hole. Denture teeth are set up on the articulated casts.

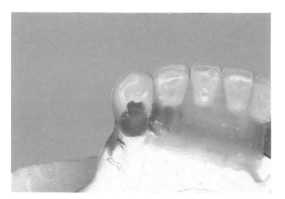

Fig. 15-19d   Plastic denture teeth are trimmed to fit close to the spacer. When adequate room exists, porcelain teeth may be used if desired.

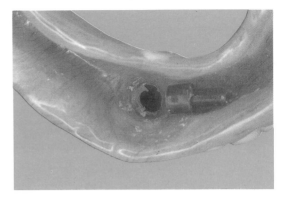

Fig. 15-19e   The spacer processed in the denture is removed to leave a formed recess. This recess is to receive the hub of the white male post. It may be necessary to enlarge this recess when the male is locked into the overdenture directly in the mouth.

into the females. Snap the white nylon male, with its centering sleeve, into the cemented female until a definite snap is felt (Fig. 15-20a). The centering sleeve must be firmly seated into the female. This sleeve serves to position the male in proper alignment to engage the female undercut and prevents acrylic resin from entering the female.

13. Insert the denture to be certain it sits passively over the male hub. If it does not, trim the hub or enlarge the male recess inside the overdenture until it does sit passively.

14. Remove the denture. With a small brush paint a small amount of self-curing acrylic resin around and particularly under the protruding male hub (Fig. 15-20b).

15. Place a small amount of resin into the recess in the tissue side of the overdenture (Fig. 15-20c).

16. Carefully insert the denture into position. The patient should be instructed to gently close into occlusion and to hold this position until the acrylic resin hardens. Thus, the male is processed in place by the self-curing resin with the denture in occlusion.

17. After the acrylic has cured, remove the overdenture, trim excess flash, and remove the centering sleeves. The overdenture is now ready for use (Fig. 15-20d).

Indirect Procedure Using Gold Copings

The Zest female can also be fabricated into a gold coping, should the dentist desire full-root coverage (Fig. 15-21). Briefly, the abutments are prepared to receive a short coping with a recess for the Zest female. During the coping wax-up technique, insert a special Zest female mounted on a ceramic rod into the die recess. As the pattern is waxed directly against the female and cast as one unit, the finished coping has the preformed female locked within it. The ceramic rod is removed with a sharp instrument. This leaves a metal coping with the female locked in position.

Gold Coping Procedure

1. Prepare the endodontically treated roots to receive a gold casting. Create a small chamfer or feather margin (Fig. 15-22a).

2. Prepare a recess three to four millimeters deep and three to four millimeters wide to receive the female (Fig. 15-22b). Use the female on the ceramic rod as a guide. If added coping retention is desired, prepare the canal for a dowel or parallel pins (Fig. 15-22c).

3. Take an impression of the prepared roots and ridge area, as you would for any crown and bridge preparation.

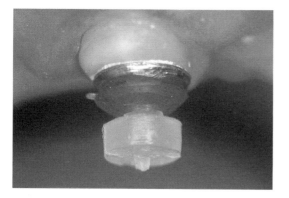

Fig. 15-20a   White male posts snapped inside the females in the mouth. The centering sleeve is forced into the female, thus positioning the male with its ball engaging the female undercut.

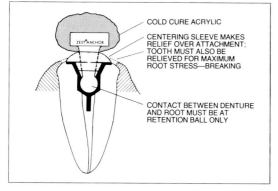

COLD CURE ACRYLIC

CENTERING SLEEVE MAKES RELIEF OVER ATTACHMENT; TOOTH MUST ALSO BE RELIEVED FOR MAXIMUM ROOT STRESS—BREAKING

CONTACT BETWEEN DENTURE AND ROOT MUST BE AT RETENTION BALL ONLY

Fig. 15-20b   Pink auto-polymerizing resin is painted around and under the hub.

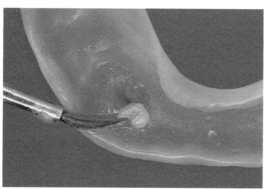

Fig. 15-20c   A very small amount of resin is placed into the prepared recess. The denture is inserted and the patient instructed to close into occlusion until the resin hardens.

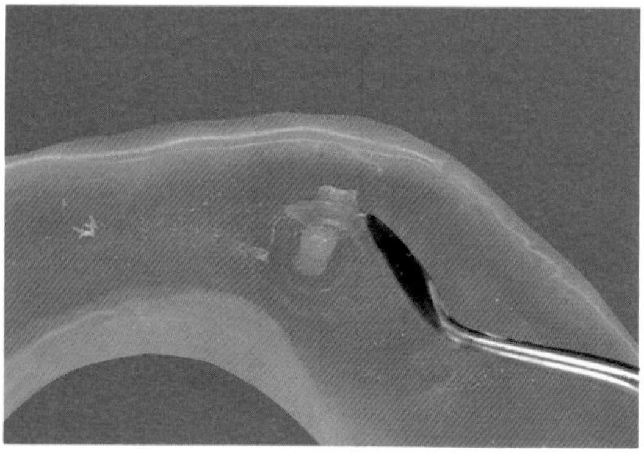

Fig. 15-20d   The excess resin and centering sleeve are removed. The overdenture is ready for insertion.

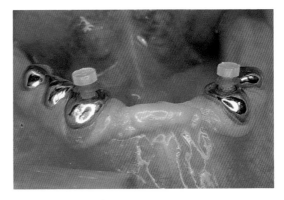

Fig. 15-21 Female Zest incorporated into a short coping. The metal female becomes an integral part of the casting.

4. Pour the impression to produce a cast with removable dies on which to fabricate the castings. Trim and lubricate the dies for waxing purposes.
5. The rods with the female should be waxed approximately parallel to each other, and to the path of insertion. The female portion should be inserted into the die recess (Fig. 15-22d). The shoulder, or surface of the metal female on the ceramic rod, should be even with the surface of the wax pattern (Fig. 15-22e).
6. Sprue the wax pattern, invest and cast.
7. The ceramic rod, which is retained within the casting, is drilled out or removed with a sharp instrument. The retentive female is retained within the casting (Fig. 15-22f). Now the polished casting is ready for cementation.
8. The males are now inserted and the treatment is similar to the techniques just discussed (Fig. 15-23).

Mini-Zest Anchorage (Fig. 15-24)

The mini-Zest is smaller than the regular Zest, being approximately 3.25 millimeters in length. Because of this, it is often more applicable in the following situations:

1. It should be used with smaller diameter roots, such as upper laterals, some bi-cuspid roots, lower anteriors, and in the pulp chamber of multi-rooted teeth (Fig. 15-25).
2. It may also be used when the pulpal chamber of teeth is very divergent from the path of insertion.

Procedures

The same step-by-step procedures discussed for the standard Zest anchor apply to the mini-Zest, with these exceptions:

1. When making the first preparation into the root with a number two bur, you need not follow the pulpal chamber.
2. The depth of this penetration need only be approximately four millimeters.
3. After widening this initial depth preparation with a fissure bur, use the mini-diamond sizing bur to prepare the seat for the female attachment.
4. Undercut the lateral wall of the recess at its base to give a more definite cement-locking effect.
5. The red substitute female must be shortened to fit the mini-female. This reduction must be made until the substitute female snaps snugly over the male extruding from the impression material. (The authors prefer using the actual mini-female instead of the substitute female).

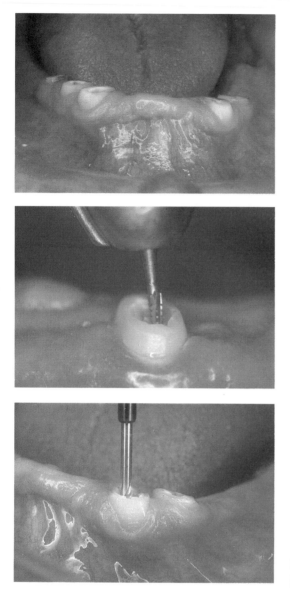

Fig. 15-22a   Endodontically treated roots prepared to receive a short coping.

Fig. 15-22b   A recess is cut into the canal with a carbide fissure bur approximately three millimeters deep and three millimeters wide. The prepared root recess is tested for available space with the metal female on its ceramic rod.

Fig. 15-22c   A dowel preparation can be prepared for additional retention.

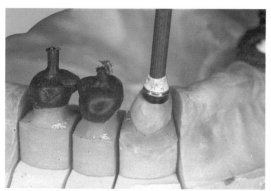

Fig. 15-22d   The ceramic rod held in a surveyor is positioned in the die space. The rod is held parallel to the path of insertion.

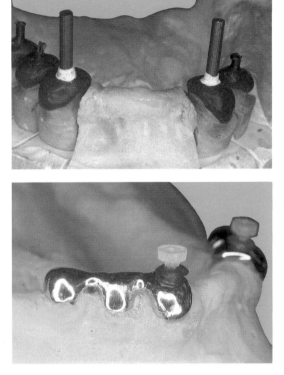

Fig. 15-22e   The female is waxed in the pattern with its diaphragm flush with the surface of the coping pattern. It is sprued, invested and cast.

Fig. 15-22f   The ceramic rod is removed with a sharp instrument, and the cast is polished and ready for insertion.

6. The same centering sleeves are used with the mini-system, though they do not position the male quite as accurately as when used with the longer female.

Relining and Rebasing Procedures

Since the purpose of the alveolar ridge is to retain the natural dentition, resorption is inevitable when teeth are removed. The patient will soon observe a torquing of the denture as the prosthesis rocks over the abutments. The more recent the extractions, the sooner the overdenture becomes unstable. Such torquing will cause severe damage to the remaining supporting abutments, if the problem is not corrected. Unstable overdentures must be relined or rebased.

The authors prefer to rebase rather than simply reline. Rebasing replaces all of the denture base material, retaining only the existing denture teeth.

Rebasing Procedures

1. If severe undercuts are present in the overdenture, trim the inside of the denture flange sufficiently to remove these undercuts.
2. Remove all male attachments and ream out additional denture base to provide room for impression material and new Zest males.
3. Place blue transfer posts into the females. The males should be accurately positioned with the centering sleeves, as described earlier.
4. Reposition the denture in the mouth to assure that the denture sits passively

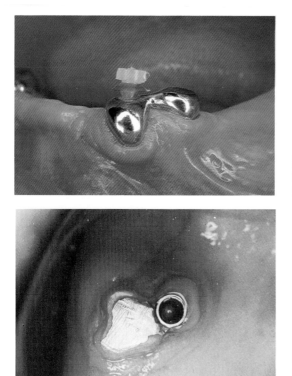

Fig. 15-23   Coping with its female cemented on the abutment. The white nylon male is inserted, ready for incorporation into the denture base.

Fig. 15-24   The mini-Zest female in a molar. The mini-Zest is approximately 3.25 millimeters and fits ideally into smaller roots.

over the male posts. If not, remove additional acrylic resin over each post, or trim the hub of the males.

5. Remove the denture, dry it thoroughly and then paint an adhesive material inside the overdenture. Take a relining impression with the material of your choice. Have the patient ease gently into occlusion as you border-mold the denture by muscle-trimming.

6. When the impression material sets, remove the denture. The male posts will be retained within the impression material.

7. Place transfer females over each male.

8. Pour the impression with stone material and trim the harden cast base.

9. Accurately mount the cast with the retained overdenture in a relining jig, as you would any conventional relining procedure. Separate the relining jig, leaving the incisal and occlusal teeth imprint in the upper member, and the cast on the lower member.

10. Remove the cast from the jig and pry off the overdenture. Remove the denture teeth and insert them in their respective plaster indexes.

11. Place white Zest males into the transfer females locked in the master model. Position the centering sleeve and block out all root undercuts with plaster.

12. Reposition the cast on the relining jig and close the jig with the teeth in position. Trim the male hub if it hits against any denture teeth. Wax the teeth into position. Wax-up the denture base and complete the overdenture, as described earlier.

13. The rebased denture is now ready for insertion.

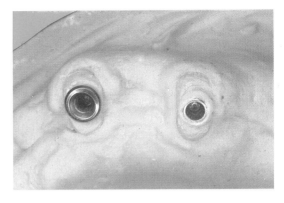

Fig. 15-25   Mini-Zest in a bicuspid. The mini-Zest is an excellent attachment modification for molars where danger of pulpal floor penetration exists.

Replacement of Broken Male Posts

Anything man-made will eventually wear or even break. This applies to the nylon male post of the Zest anchor. With normal usage, wear is not excessive; however, it can become a problem under certain conditions.

Often when the soft or bony tissue undercuts are excessive, it is difficult for the patient to accurately insert the overdenture. Here, insertion will cause excessive flexing of the male and thus encourage breakage. Occasionally the patient will develop a habit of biting the overdenture in place. This is a bad habit since the chances of breaking male posts are increased.

Excessive breakage, or premature wear of the male posts, is usually due to specific causes; for example: poor occlusion, overextended denture flanges, misaligned females, an inaccurately fitting overdenture, or where the alveolar process has resorbed excessively. Replacing the male posts should not be done without correcting the cause of the excessive wear; otherwise, breakage will continue.

Replacing the males

1. Remove the male post from the denture base. Remove additional acrylic to provide room for the new male post.
2. Insert a white male into the female.
3. Insert the overdenture to be sure that it fits passively over the male.
4. Remove the overdenture and the male post.
5. Place a small amount of Vaseline into the female, insert the male firmly into place. Align the male by firmly seating the centering sleeve. Then remove any excess Vaseline.
6. Place a small amount of self-curing resin around and under the hub of the male post and a minimal amount into the overdenture recess.
7. Insert the overdenture and have the patient close lightly into occlusion until the acrylic resin cures.
8. Remove the overdenture from the mouth. Remove the centering sleeve and any excess acrylic flash. The overdenture is now ready for insertion.

Miscellaneous Uses for the Zest

The Zest anchor can also be used with overlay partial dentures, permitting teeth that would otherwise be sacrificed to function as supporting or retentive abutments.

Trouble-shooting with Zest Anchor

The Zest also may be used directly with previously constructed copings where other attachments have failed under an overdenture. To trouble-shoot such a failure with a Zest anchor, follow these procedures:

1. Drill pilot holes through the castings with a number four round bur being careful not to drill into the root. Continue with a number two round bur into the root, approximately six millimeters.
2. Enlarge the hole in the casting with a carbide fissure bur to receive the diamond sizing bur.
3. Use the carbide fissure bur to flatten and parallel the occlusal surface of the copings to receive the flat area of the diamond bur. This will minimize the drilling that is necessary with the diamond sizing bur to produce the female recess.
4. Cement the female into the casting as you would an inlay. The Zest anchor will also provide retention for the coping, acting as a post.
5. Insert the nylon males into the females and process into the previously constructed denture, as described earlier.

Chapter 16

Bar Attachments

As the name suggests, bar attachments consist of a metal bar that splints two or more abutments, and a companion mechanism processed within the tissue area of the overdenture (Fig. 16-1). This mechanism snaps on the bar to retain the prosthesis.

Bar attachments are available commercially in a wide variety of forms or they can easily be "custom" fabricated.

Whether a bar system is best for a particular prosthesis depends upon several considerations.

1. Will the overdenture be supported by abutments with short copings?
2. Will the overdenture be supported by abutments with long copings?
3. Will the abutments provide support and stability in more than one plane?
4. How much retention is needed?
5. Splinting weak abutments?
6. Should the abutments support most (or very little) of the masticating load?
7. Personal preference.

Types of Bar Attachments

There are numerous modifications of bar attachments available to provide excellent splinting and retention action. However, there are two basic types based on the shape and action performed; bar units and bar joints (Figs. 16-2a and b).

The Bar Unit

This bar has parallel walls providing rigid fixation with frictional retention. It can be used for retention with long, medium or short copings, but only when the appliance is to be an all-tooth-supported appliance (i.e. where no stress-broken or rotational action is indicated). It is never used when a bar joint is indicated (when rotational or vertical action is necessary); however, a bar joint can be used whenever a bar unit is indicated.

The Bar Joint

The action of this attachment provides rotational or vertical movement. In other words, it is a stress-broken attachment. It has a rounded or semi-rounded contour so the retention clip and prosthesis can rotate slightly during mastication (Fig. 16-3).

Bar joints are excellent attachments when used under these conditions:

Like the bar unit, the bar joint splints the abutments, retains, supports and stabilizes the overdenture. And like the bar unit, it can be used with long, medium or short copings. However, unlike the bar unit, a bar joint minimizes forces on the abutments through its stress-broken rotation. Since the typical overdenture abutment is extremely weak, the bar joint is generally preferred to the bar unit.

When two abutments, such as two cuspids, are splinted, the overdenture is supported in

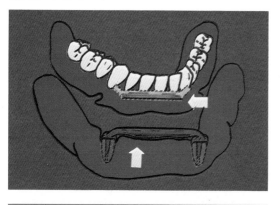

Fig. 16-1 A bar fixation splints two or more abutments stabilizing the weak abutments and providing retention for the overdenture. The overdenture fixation is obtained when a retentive shell, or clip (processed in the denture base), engages the bar.

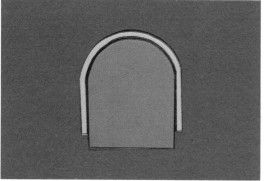

Fig. 16-2a The Dolder bar unit has a "U-shaped" configuration. When its parallel walls are engaged by the retentive shell, a rigid fixation is obtained. Such an anchorage system does not provide for any rotational or vertical movement of the overdenture.

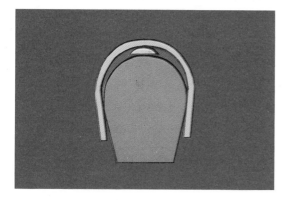

Fig. 16-2b Bar joint has a general rounded shape that permits some degree of overdenture movement. This movement may be a vertical and rotational movement, or just a rotational action. Notice the spacer over the bar which is removed after overdenture fabrication.

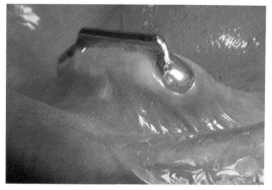

Fig. 16-3 A common application of the bar fixation splinting two lower cuspids with a Dolder bar joint. The retention and stability are in one plane.

one plane. When more than two weaker abutments are present in one plane, the abutment copings may be splinted with a bar but stability is still provided in just one plane. When an additional abutment is present posteriorly, support would be much improved by providing stability in two planes (Fig. 16-4). In fact, if two strong abutments are present in one plane, stability can be increased by cantilevering one or even two short bars distally to the abutments to create stability in two or three planes (see Fig. 2-3c). When another abutment is present posteriorly in the opposite quadrant, the abutments are now in three planes (Fig. 16-5). This provides maximum support, stability and retention.

The Dolder Bar

An ideal bar attachment is the Dolder bar (Fig. 16-3). It is well-designed for splinting two or more abutments to provide support, stability and retention for the overdenture. This bar attachment is manufactured in two forms – a bar joint and a bar unit, shown from left to right (Fig. 16-6). It is also available in two different diameters and lengths.

a) The pear-shaped bar joint is designed to provide vertical and rotational action so it is indicated where a stress-broken, resilient attachment is desired. It can also be used as a bar unit for an all-tooth-supported prosthesis by fabricating the overdenture without planned vertical movement.

b) The bar unit is in the form of an inverted U with parallel walls. It does not permit rotational or vertical movement; therefore it only provides retention and support, but maximizes the masticatory load on the abutments.

Typical Dolder Bar Treatment

The following condition illustrates a common application of the resilient Dolder bar attachment. This patient, a sixty-nine-year-old female, had six remaining lower anterior teeth (Fig. 16-7). The cuspids were retained to be splinted by the bar and the central and lateral incisors were removed. The patient was treated in this manner:

1. Endodontics, extractions and periodontal surgery were completed prior to starting the operative process (see "Treatment Planning," Chapter 3). Tooth preparations were started only after healing.
2. With a carbide or diamond fissure bur mounted in a high-speed handpiece, reduce the endodontically treated cuspids to one to two millimeters above the gingiva (Fig. 16-8).
3. Now use a diamond bur to prepare the abutments with a bevel or chamfer margin.
4. An X indentation was cut into the occlusal surface of each root with an inverted cone bur or with the corner of a flat end diamond bur (see Fig. 8-6). The strength of the coping diaphragm is increased by the added thickness provided by the indentation. The thinner the coping diaphragm the better the crown-root ratio.
5. Retention of the gold casting on the root is an important consideration. Short copings have minimal frictional retention so some auxiliary coping retention is imperative. The copings can be retained with posts, parallel or non-parallel pins, or a combination of both. As the two cuspids will be splinted with the bar joint, the posts (used in this case) must be parallel to each other. The para-post system with the Para-Max (See "Coping Retention," chapter 8), was used to prepare these parallel "sized" holes to receive the impression posts (see Fig. 9-8).
6. Enlarge the canal opening with a number six or eight bur to one half of the bur head depth (see Fig. 9-9). This adds strength to the dowel-casting union here.
7. Fabricate a customized impression tray on the study cast. Prepare holes in the

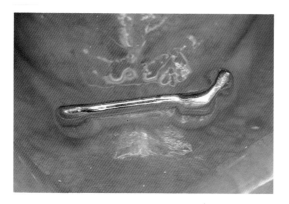

Fig. 16-4 Overdenture stability, support and retention increased by adding another abutment distally. In such a situation, stability is in two planes; one anterior and one posterior.

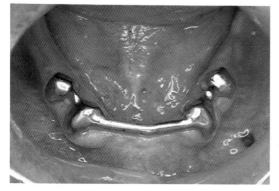

Fig. 16-5 Three-plane stability with anterior abutments and bilateral posterior abutments splinted with bar anchorage. Such three-plane arrangements provide ideal stability and retention.

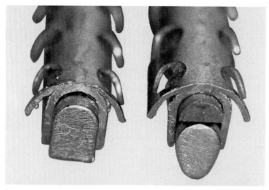

Fig. 16-6 The Dolder bar is available as a bar joint (with a "pear-shaped" configuration) that accommodates movement of the prosthesis; and a bar unit (with a "U-shape") providing only rigid fixation. The retentive shell of the bar joint is separated by a spacer. No spacer is supplied with the bar unit. The retentive shell has a special perforated mechanical retention.

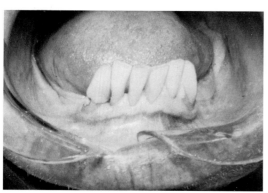

Fig. 16-7 A sixty-nine-year-old female patient with six remaining anterior teeth. The two cuspids are going to be retained and their copings splinted with a Dolder bar attachment.

tray over the root preparations (see Fig. 10-1e). The impression posts will pass through these holes.

8. Take a muscle-trimmed impression of the teeth and soft tissue areas. The previously positioned impression posts are withdrawn with the impression (see Fig. 10-3).

9. The impression is poured in stone to produce a master cast with removable dies. Before removing the impression from the cast, carefully remove the impression material over the impression posts (see Fig. 10-4).

10. Gently remove the impression posts with a hemostat before removing the master cast from the impression (see Fig. 10-5). This will eliminate any danger of fracturing the stone dies.

11. Trim the dies of the master cast, place plastic posts in the dies, shorten the posts and flatten them with a hot spatula (Fig. 16-9). These posts should extend four to five millimeters beyond the dowel canal opening.

12. Lubricate the dies and wax the patterns for short copings (Fig. 16-10) (see "Coping Form," chapters 4 and 11).

13. Sprue, invest and cast the copings. The copings are finished, but are left with a short section of the sprue on each casting which will be removed later. These retained sprue posts aid in the assembly of the bar to the copings for soldering (Fig. 16-11).

14. Mount the casts on an articulator with appropriate intra-occlusal records obtained with custom trays and wax occlusal rims.

15. Set up the denture teeth and check with the patient for occlusal harmony, vertical dimension and esthetics (Fig. 16-12).

16. Cut the bar to fit between the copings. The bar should be positioned slightly lingual to allow room for the anterior teeth but not too far to interfere with tongue action (Fig. 16-13). If the bar is positioned too far labially, the anteriorly

positioned teeth will give the lower lip a very poor esthetic appearance.

Adapt the bar closely to the crest of the alveolar ridge by grinding the gingival portion. The bar should also be positioned horizontally. When the arch is tapering, either bend the bar or cut and solder the bar to conform to the curvature of the arch.

17. To aid in orienting the bar correctly, the previously set-up anterior teeth can be indexed with a plaster core.

18. Connect the bar to the copings (the short sprue stubs help here) with Duralay, or sticky wax. Invest and solder to the copings. Polish the substructure and place on the master cast for assembly (Fig. 16-14).

19. Retention of the overlay prosthesis is provided by the retentive shell processed in the tissue side of the denture base. Cut the shell to fit against the proximal surface of each coping (Fig. 16-15). This retentive shell is fabricated with perforated wings, to lock the clip into the denture base. The authors have experienced much breakage of these spot-welded resin retention flanges. The shorter the retentive shell, the more likely the breakage. Therefore, the following modification is recommended (Figs. 16-16a and b):

a) Remove the retentive flanges, or bend them completely over.
b) Cut a small section from the corner of each flange.
c) Bend up each free end section to form a definite lug for retention in the denture base resin.
d) For an exceptionally long attachment, cut two slits midway in each flange. The resultant sections are then bent upward to produce additional retentive lugs.
e) Often it is helpful to cut numerous slits into the flanges. Later, individual sections can be adjusted for retention (Fig. 16-17).

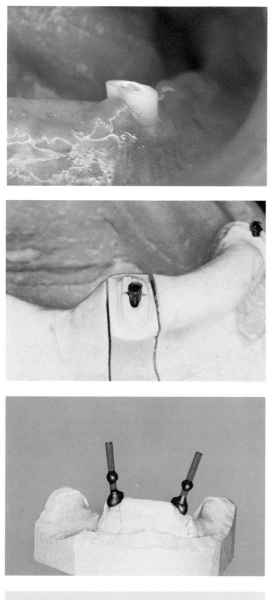

Fig. 16-8   Two cuspid abutments prepared to receive Dolder bar-splinted short copings. The initial preparation is made by sectioning through the crown with a fissure bur one to two millimeters above the gingiva. The root surface follows closely the contour of the alveolar ridge.

Fig. 16-9   Plastic dowels used as the dowel pattern. First, flatten the end of each plastic dowel pattern with a hot spatula. The wax pattern will be more securely fastened to this flattened area. The dowels can also be left long and used as the pattern sprue when fitted with a reservoir.

Fig. 16-10   Short coping patterns are waxed to conform to the curvature of the alveolar ridge. Such an arrangement produces a coping with the most favorable crown-root ratio, and space for the set-up of the denture teeth.

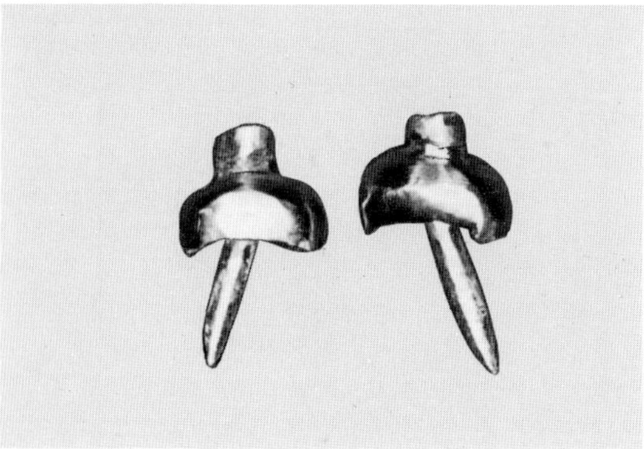

Fig. 16-11   A short section of sprue is retained on each coping. The sprue stubs help to secure the copings to the bar for soldering. These stubs also help to lock the coping in an impression when a master impression is taken with the castings seated on the abutments.

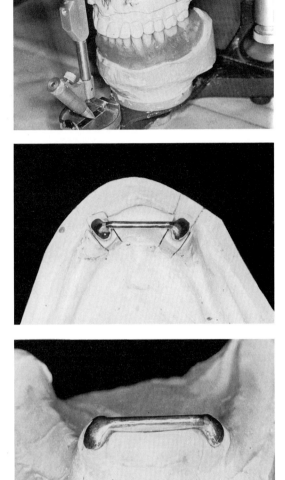

Fig. 16-12 The master cast with its copings is mounted on an appropriate articulator and the denture teeth set up. This initial denture set-up may aid in the positioning of the bar. The anterior teeth may be indexed with a plaster core to aid in the bar location.

Fig. 16-13 Position the bar slightly lingual to the crest of the ridge. This generally allows adequate room for the anterior teeth, but still not too far lingual to interfere with the tongue. It should be positioned horizontally and in light contact with the alveolar ridge. Often, it may be necessary to bend, or cut and solder, the bar to conform to the ridge curvature.

Fig. 16-14 Copings soldered to the Dolder bar. The copings were positioned on their dies and locked to the bar with Duralay, invested and then soldered to produce this dowel-retained coping-bar substructure. The soldered joint, gingivally, should not interfere with the gingival tissue. This joint should be opened to form a definite gingival embrasure where the bar joins the coping.

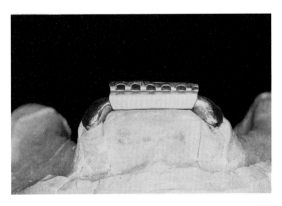

Fig. 16-15 The retentive shell cut to fit over the bar and against the proximal surface of each coping. The edges of the shell should be flush to the coping wall to help prevent lateral shifting of the overdenture.

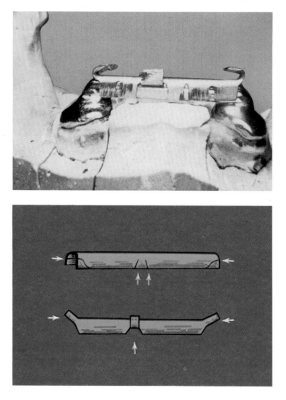

Fig. 16-16a A shell modified for better resin retention. Retentive lugs bent into the retentive shell will produce a more definite "lock" in the denture base.

Fig. 16-16b The retentive shell can be modified for a more secure lock into the denture base: first, remove a small section from the corner of the flanges. Next, bend up the remaining portion to produce a retentive lug. For a long retentive shell, make two cuts into each flange. Then bend up the wings produce by these cuts.

20. The metal spacer is positioned over the bar and the retentive shell is snapped on the bar securing the spacer (Fig. 16-18). Since this Dolder bar joint is a resilient attachment, when the spacer is removed later, the prosthesis will be spaced for vertical movement.

21. Space must also be provided over the copings. This space over the copings and between the denture base is provided in this manner: before the denture teeth are set up, three to four thicknesses of X-ray foil are adapted over each coping (Fig. 16-19). All spacers will be removed after the overdenture is processed.

22. Block out all undercuts around the copings with plaster and cover the flanges of the retentive shell (Fig. 16-20). If this is not done properly, acrylic resin processed against the shell will prevent the female

retentive areas from flexing. This will eliminate its retentive action.

In addition, it is of utmost importance that this blocking-out process not be excessive. Otherwise, spaces between the denture base and soft tissues will be left where gingival tissue may proliferate (Fig. 16-21).

23. With a small brush, sparingly paint a semi-dry mix of auto-polymerizing acrylic resin (such as Duralay) to cover the end of the spacer and shell (Fig. 16-22). This prevents processed denture acrylic being forced into this space locking the bar and shell assembly together. Placing plaster here is often ineffective. Often this plaster will be dislodged during the denture packing process. Now, processed resin will lock the coping-bar assembly to the overdenture. The prosthesis

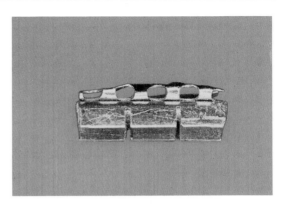

Fig. 16-17 Slits cut into the flanges of a long shell. Variability in retention can be modified more effectively by bending each individual clasp section for a uniform control of retention.

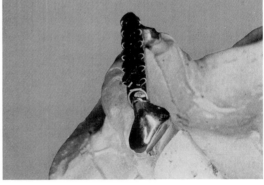

Fig. 16-18 Retentive shell with spacer positioned over the bar. An overdenture designed to be "resilient" must be fabricated with the substructure spaced.

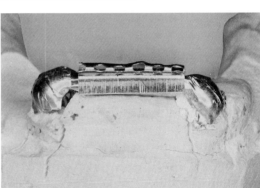

Fig. 16-19 Closely adapt three to four thicknesses of X-ray foil over each coping and position the spacer on the bar. After the prosthesis is fabricated and these spacers are removed, a space will exist between the tissue side of the denture base, the inside of the retentive shell, and the coping-bar substructure. This space will be the thickness of the foil and spacer and will provide rotational and vertical movement.

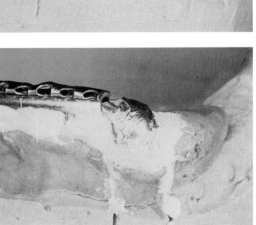
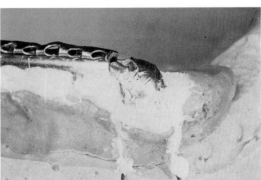

Fig. 16-20 Undercuts around the copings blocked out with plaster. A minimum of plaster should be used. The retentive flanges of the shell must also be covered with a minimum of plaster. Excess blocking-out with plaster is a frequent reason for overdenture problems from formation of air space and tissue proliferation.

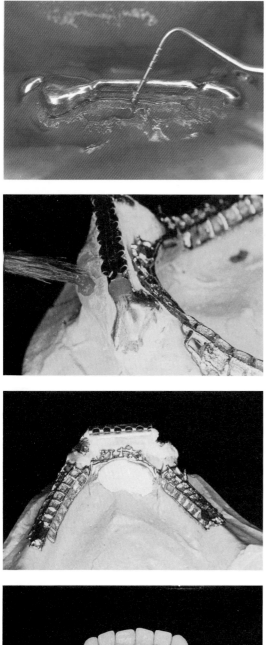

Fig. 16-21 Proliferation of gingival tissue around a bar attachment into excess space produced by extensive blocking-out procedures.

Fig. 16-22 Duralay was used to cover only the open ends of the shell and spacer. This resin is not as easily dislodged during overdenture fabrication as is plaster. This prevents the possibility of the retentive shell (and overdenture) being locked to the coping-bar assembly. The Duralay should be a firm mix and not soupy, otherwise it will flow over the bar and copings, locking the overdenture to the substructure.

Fig. 16-23 The framework is locked in position on the cast with plaster to prevent its dislodgement during the overdenture flasking process. The reinforcing framework was designed with a short lingual bar major connector and a simple mesh for securing the denture base. This framework, however, can be designed with the overdenture flange partially or completely in metal.

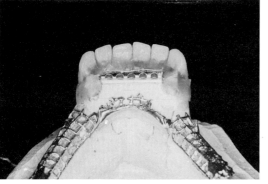

Fig. 16-24 Anterior teeth are repositioned with the plaster index. Any interfering "blocking-out" plaster is carefully removed until the anteriors seat accurately. Examine these areas and replace any plaster inadvertently removed from the undercuts.

may be damaged while removing this resin. Occasionally the coping-bar assembly may even be bent.

24. Although an overdenture without strengthening framework may be constructed, the authors recommend that all overlay dentures be reinforced. Most dentures without such a reinforcement eventually fracture (Fig. 16-23) (see "Framework Design," chapter 12). The framework is locked on the cast with plaster.

25. Use the stone index to reposition the anterior teeth and complete the denture set-up (Fig. 16-24). Be certain that the blocking-out plaster does not interfere with positive seating of the anterior teeth. Trim any of the plaster that may interfere with the positioning of the denture set-up.

26. The denture is waxed, festooned, flasked, processed and finished. The coping-bar assembly is removed but the retentive shell is retained within the tissue side of the denture (Fig. 16-25a). The lead foil, and auxiliary spacer, as well as any excess acrylic is carefully removed (Fig. 16-25b).

27. Cement the Dolder bar/coping assembly into position. The overlay denture is inserted for use (Fig. 16-26).

Overdenture Function

Let us now consider the function of this overdenture. Freedom for vertical movement, provided by the auxiliary wire spacer and lead foil covering the copings during fabrication, allows approximately 0.5 to 1.0 millimeter of space for movement during function (Fig. 16-27a). At rest, the overdenture sits passively only on the alveolar tissues. A space is present between the bar-coping assembly and the shell-tissue side of the overdenture. There is maximum retention now since the clip engages the bar undercut (Fig. 16-27b).

During mastication, the denture moves verti-

cally. Now it is supported by both the alveolar tissues and the root supported coping-bar substructure. No space is present over the bar and copings. The abutment teeth and soft tissue now absorb maximum denture function (Fig. 16-27c).

When the supporting tissue is thin, as in the lower arch, the tissue can be compressed only slightly before the prosthesis should rest on the coping-bar substructure. Approximately 0.5 millimeter space should be provided in this situation. On the more spongy, fibrous resilient tissues, tissue compression is generally greater. A space of approximately one millimeter may be required now.

Adjusting Retention

Retention of the overdenture is easily increased or decreased by adjusting the flanges of the shell to provide desirable retention.

Bending the lingual flange will depress the distal base of the denture. Bending the labial flange tends to keep the anterior segment down. These adjustments can be made easily by inserting a sharp instrument between the retentive blades and the denture base and applying slight pressure to bend the flange. This retention should not be excessive, otherwise excess stresses will be subjected to the substructure and abutments.

Relining/Rebasing Technique

As the alveolar ridge resorbs, the overdenture settles and rocks on the Dolder bar assembly. These excessive masticatory loads direct damaging torquing stresses to the abutments. When this occurs, the following rebasing procedure should be followed.

1. With a small round bur, carefully remove the acrylic around the shell, and remove the shell. It will be used later.
2. Remove additional acrylic above the area of the copings and bar using a straight

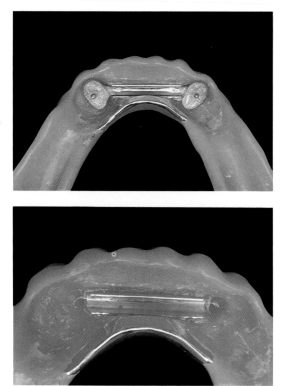

Fig. 16-25a   The coping-bar assembly locked inside the overdenture. It is removed carefully with all spacers and any excess resin that may interfere with the insertion of the prosthesis. If the assembly cannot be removed, processed resin may have been inadvertently processed around the bar or copings. Force should not be used, otherwise the bar may be bent. Use a small bur to carefully remove the offending resin. Careful blocking out with plaster is very important for this reason.

Fig. 16-25b   The retentive shell exposed in the overdenture. Any resin processed against the retentive lamellae must be removed to free the lamellae to act as a clasping device.

handpiece with a number eight bur. This additional space will accommodate the impression material.

3. Dry the denture and paint the tissue areas with an impression adhesive.

4. Using the elastic impression material of your choice, take an impression of the tissue-bearing areas, copings and Dolder bar. The patient should close gently into occlusion, as you muscle-trim the impression material. When a large space is present under the bar or between the copings, it should be blocked out with soft wax or cement prior to taking the impression. Otherwise, tearing-away of the impression material from these voids, when the impression is removed, will distort and destroy the accuracy of fit when the prosthesis is rebased.

5. The impression is poured with model stone.

6. The cast with the overdenture attached is mounted in a relining jig. The teeth are indexed in the opposing member and the jig is opened after the plaster has set.

7. The overdenture is removed from the cast ieaving a reproduction of the soft tissue, the copings and Dolder bar (Fig. 16-28a).

8. The denture teeth are removed from the overdenture and are positioned in their appropriate slot in the plaster index. These teeth may be secured with a very small drop of sticky wax.

9. The cast is now treated as if you are fabricating a new overdenture (Fig. 16-28b), i. e.,

   a) Place three to four layers of X-ray foil over each coping as a spacer.

   b) Place the metal spacer over the mold of the bar.

Fig. 16-26 Before cementing the coping-bar assembly, test the fit of the copings on the abutments. Insert the overdenture over the bar substructure to test its fit and function. If insertion difficulty is experienced, carefully examine the inside of the denture base and remove any interfering resin. Free the lamellae of any resin that may need removing. Cement the substructure with "crown and bridge" cement and remove all excess cement when hardened. When the overdenture is inserted, it should be adjusted for a "loose" fit until the cement has hardened sufficiently. Otherwise, the overdenture may loosen the freshly cemented substructure.

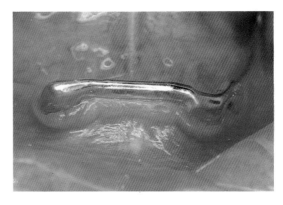

c) Snap the retentive shell into position over the spacer and plaster bar.
d) Using plaster, block out the retentive flanges of the shell and all undercuts.
e) Block the ends of the shell and spacer with resin.
f) Reposition the cast on the relining jig; wax the teeth into position; wax the denture base; festoon, flask, pack, cure and finish the overdenture as in any complete denture technique.
g) The rebased overdenture is now ready for insertion.

The Dolder Bar Unit

The Dolder bar unit is an excellent attachment when an all-tooth-supported, non-rotational acting overdenture is desired (see Fig. 16-2). This bar design may be indicated if there are numerous abutments – especially if they are located in three planes; i.e. posterior and anterior abutments (Fig. 16-29).
As mentioned earlier, the bar unit is not rounded like the bar joint, but rather has parallel walls. The friction between these walls and the shell provides the retention. Like the bar joint, the Dolder Unit is available in two sizes. The larger has a vertical bar dimension of four to five millimeters. The smaller, a vertical dimension of 3.6 millimeters.

Because the bar unit has parallel walls, the female shell does not flex much during insertion. This means that the unit leaves less open space than the joint where tissue may proliferate. This is a decided advantage. Of course, it can be used only where no rotational overdenture function occurs.

General Technique

The bar unit fabrication technique is virtually the same as that using the bar joint but with these exceptions:

1. No spacer is placed over the bar. The clasping shell fits directly on the bar.
2. No spacing is necessary over the copings.
3. Parallelism of the bar is more critical than with the Dolder bar joint.
4. A special paralleling mandrel is used to parallel the bar unit.

Other Bar Systems

The dentist is not limited to the Dolder bar joint or unit. There are many other bar systems available commercially, such as the Hader bar, Octalink, Ceka, Ackerman, M.F. Channels and C.M. Bars. In addition, bars can be "customized," using a variety of tech-

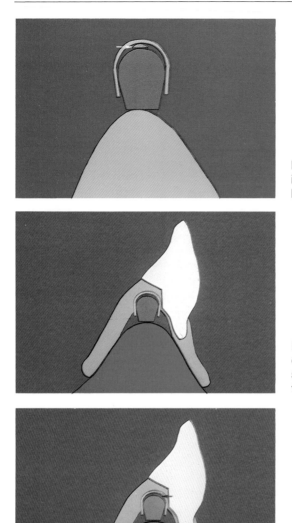

Fig. 16-27a   Dolder bar function: With the spacer in place there is maximum retention with the lamellae engaging the bar "undercut."

Fig. 16-27b   With the spacer removed and the denture resting passively on the tissues, there is a space over the bar and coping (the thickness of the spacer). Maximum retention is present.

Fig. 16-27c   During function, there will be no space over the bar, or copings, with maximum tissue and abutment support present.

niques. Commercial retentive clips can be used with these customized bars.

Customized Bars

As the overall treatment using bar-retained overdentures has been thoroughly discussed, we shall consider only customization of the bar and utilization of the reten-

tive clasp. The overall clinical and laboratory use of customized bars varies little from the important basic technique used with the Dolder bar system.

Round Wax Patterns

Round spruing wax makes an excellent pattern for bar fabrication (Fig. 16-30). After the

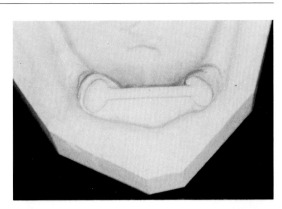

Fig. 16-28a   A master cast of the coping-bar assembly and denture-bearing soft tissue, fabricated from the overdenture relining impression, readied for rebasing procedure. This cast of the copings and bar is treated as in the original fabrication techniques.

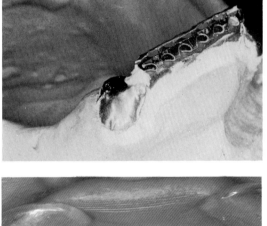

Fig. 16-28b   The copings are spaced, the shell is snapped over its spacer and the bar and undercuts blocked out with plaster. Then the denture teeth are repositioned as in any complete denture relining technique.

Fig. 16-29   The Dolder unit is indicated for an all-tooth support prosthesis. The parallel-walled bar assembly allows no freedom of overdenture movement, rotational or vertical.

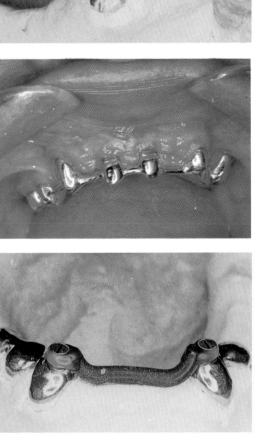

Fig. 16-30   A ten gauge sprue wax used as a pattern for a customized bar. The pattern can be adapted closely to the gingiva and bent to the curvature of the ridge.

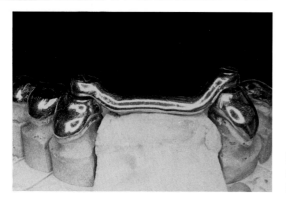

Fig. 16-31 The round-wax pattern is cast and soldered to the attachments. A Schubiger attachment was used in this situation.

coping patterns have been waxed on their respective dies, select a round wax – 8, 10 or 12 gauge in diameter. The longer the edentulous span covered, the larger the wax diameter used.

Cut a section of round wax to fit between the coping patterns. Adapt the round wax so that it contacts the alveolar tissues and conforms to the curvature of the alveolar ridge. Connect one end of the bar pattern to just one coping pattern. After the patterns have been sprued and cast, solder the bar to the other coping (Fig. 16-31). The bar pattern can also be shaped to fit the retentive clip, and then is polished ready for assembly.

Resin Patterns

Resin patterns of Dolder bar joint or unit make excellent customized patterns. In fact, you can use the Dolder joint shell itself as a mold to form a bar. The technique, which is often used by the authors, is fast and inexpensive and particularly applicable where there are irregularities in the alveolar ridge. Simply select the size shell that corresponds to the bar you wish to fabricate, and lubricate the inside with Masque or silicone spray. If a bar joint pattern is to be produced, bend the flanges together slightly. This will form a "pear-shaped" pattern. If a bar unit pattern is desired, spread the flanges so as to produce a parallel-walled resin pattern. Fill the shell with Duralay (Fig. 16-32a). After it hardens,

remove the Duralay bar and use it as a pattern (Fig. 16-32b). If there are irregularities in the ridge, add wax to the gingival portion of the resin bar pattern until the bar is in light tissue contact (Fig. 16-32c).

Since the shell is used to form the bar, a good male/female fit is virtually assured, and you can wax the bar directly to the copings for a one-piece casting.

Retentive Clips Used with Customized Bars

Numerous metal clips are available to fit customized bars: Ackerman clip, Hader bar metal rider, Baker clip and the Dolder bar shell. These clips can be modified or adjusted to fit the bar, or the bar can be shaped to fit the retentive clip. With a ten or twelve gauge bar made from a round wax pattern, use the metal Hader rider, Ackerman or Baker clip (Fig. 16-33). If a clip normally used with a twelve gauge bar is to be used with an eight or ten gauge round customized bar, the wax bar pattern should be softened and shaped to a smaller diameter to fit the clip. Such a wax pattern can even be given a "pear-shape" (similar to a Dolder bar joint).

Of course the Dolder bar shell will fit the bar made from the Dolder shell resin pattern. It can also be modified to fit the round bars mentioned above.

The metal riders used with the Hader bar system are designed to allow rotational action

Figs. 16-32a to c Fabricating resin Dolder bar patterns.

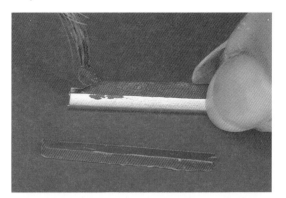

Fig. 16-32a Lubricated Dolder bar shell is filled with a mix of Duralay and the it is allowed to cure.

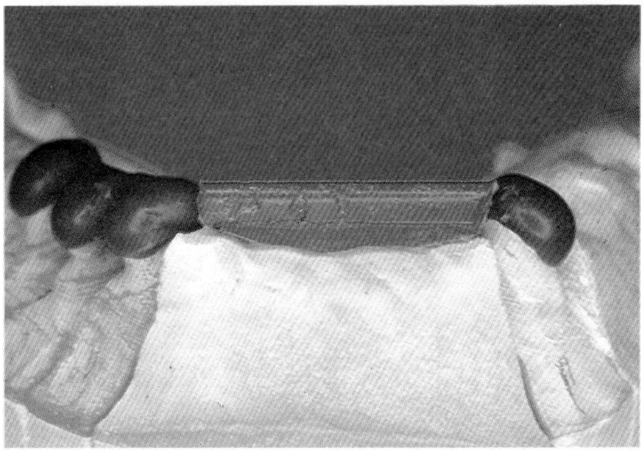

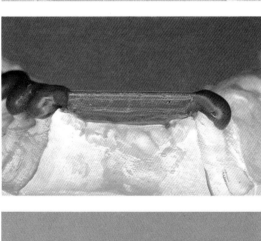

Fig. 16-32b The resin bar pattern is then removed from the shell. If the pattern is to form a bar unit, it is left as is; if it is to act as a bar joint, trim the gingival portion of the bar slightly.

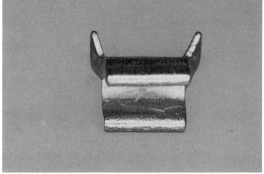

Fig. 16-32c A resin Dolder bar pattern connected to waxed coping pattern. Wax is added gingivally to adjust the pattern to differences in the gingival contour. This is a decided advantage over the metal bar.

Fig. 16-33 Ackerman clip used to provide retention with a customized round bar.

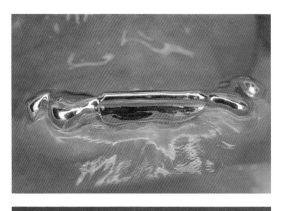

Fig. 16-34   A Hader bar anchorage splinting four abutments to provide support and retention for the overdenture. The bar was fabricated from a plastic bar pattern.

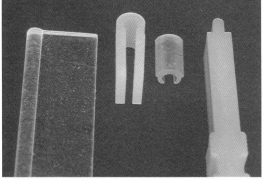

Fig. 16-35   The Hader bar system (from left to right): Plastic bar used as a pattern to fabricate a bar with parallel walls and a rounded top. A modeling rider (used in the overdenture fabricating technique) forms a preformed slot inside the denture base to receive the plastic retentive clip. A plastic retentive clip (rider), is snapped into the denture base. It will engage the rounded portion of the bar when the prosthesis is inserted. A rider seating tool is used to force the plastic rider into its preformed slot within the denture base.

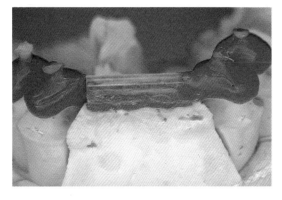

Fig. 16-36   A plastic Hader bar is cut to size and waxed to the coping patterns. The bar pattern is adjusted to fit in light contact with irregularities of the alveolar ridge. It is placed horizontal to and slightly lingual to the crest of the alveolar ridge. Its gingival length can be modified and extended to the gingiva by adding wax.

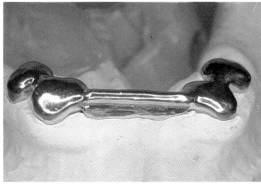

Fig. 16-37   The coping-bar assembly on the master cast. Results are improved if the assembly is first fitted on the abutments and then "pulled" with a special impression. It becomes an integral part of the new master cast for fabrication of the overlay prosthesis.

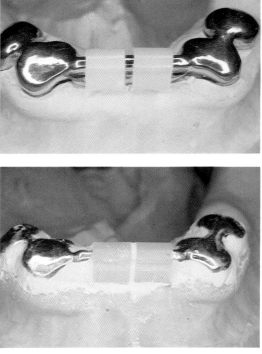

Fig. 16-38 Modeling riders in position over the Hader bar casting. This rider is positioned everywhere a retentive rider is to be inserted into the denture base. It forms a recess inside the denture base to receive the retentive rider. It is discarded after the overdenture is fabricated.

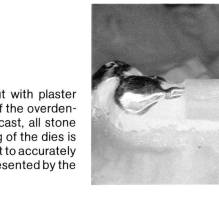

Fig. 16-39 Undercuts blocked out with plaster around the coping-bar assembly. If the overdenture is fabricated on the original cast, all stone destroyed by cutting and trimming of the dies is replaced with plaster. It is important to accurately reproduce those tissue areas represented by the cast.

without vertical translation. The disadvantage of the metal Hader rider is its lack of a sufficient retentive mechanism to hold the clip within the denture resin. The Ackerman clip is an excellent clip with pre-existing retentive wings, useful with round customized bars. The advantage of the Dolder shell is its ability to provide both rotational and vertical overdenture function.

The Hader Bar System

The Hader system is an excellent bar attachment (Fig. 16-34). Similar to the customized bar, the Hader system consists of a plastic bar pattern with gingival extension and small plastic clips that are processed into the overdenture. This system has some advantages over others; the plastic bar pattern's gingival extension can be trimmed to conform to the ridge. In addition, worn clips can be easily replaced at chairside using a special seating tool.

Components of Attachment

Components of the Hader system are (from left to right) (Fig. 16-35).
1. Plastic bar pattern (1.8 mm diameter, vertical height 5.7 mm).
2. Plastic clips (5 mm long, 3 mm thick, 4 mm high).
3. Modeling riders used in processing to create a slot for the clips.
4. Clip seating tool.

Hader Bar Technique

1. Take an impression of the prepared abutments, pour a cast and trim the dies as you would any bar-retained overdenture.

191

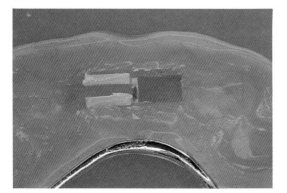

Fig. 16-40   The modeling riders retained with the denture base are removed with a hemostat or pliers. This will leave a recess similar in form to the curved slotted portion of the plastic rider.

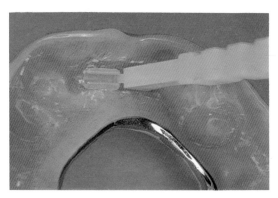

Fig. 16-41   The rider seating tool is used to insert the plastic rider into its recess preformed by the modeling rider.

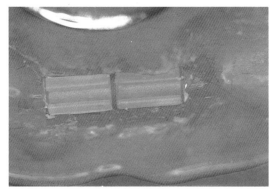

Fig. 16-42   Plastic riders locked inside the denture base. It provides retention when the overlay denture is inserted. Worn riders can easily be removed and replaced when needed. The degree of retention with the plastic rider is fixed and cannot be altered.

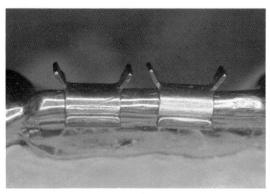

Fig. 16-43   Metal riders can be used for retention instead of the plastic riders. The authors prefer these metal riders since their retention is adjustable, whereas the plastic rider retention is fixed.

2. Wax the coping pattern on the dies.
3. Cut the bar pattern to fit between the coping patterns.
4. Heat the bar pattern and adapt it to the ridge curvature.
5. Trim the gingival portion of the bar pattern to fit the alveolar ridge.
6. Wax the plastic pattern directly to the coping patterns for a single casting, or for greater accuracy, cast separately and solder to the copings (Fig. 16-36).
7. The completed substructure pattern is sprued, invested, cast and finished.
8. Seat the substructure on the cast for completion of the overdenture (Fig. 16-37).
9. Position modeling riders on the bar where clips will attach (Fig. 16-38). These riders are removed after the prosthesis is fabricated, leaving a preformed seat to receive the plastic clips for retention.
10. Using plaster, block out all undercuts around copings and below the round portion of the bar (Fig. 16-39).
11. Set up the denture teeth, wax the denture, flask, pack and finish as for any bar overdenture technique.
12. When the overdenture is finished, remove the modeling riders with pliers or a sharp instrument (Fig. 16-40).
13. Use the special seating tool to insert the plastic clip into the slots formed by the modeling rider (Fig. 16-41). The denture is now ready for use (Fig. 16-42).

Relining/Rebasing the Hader Bar System

When relining the Hader bar overdenture, remove the plastic riders and several millimeters of acrylic over all areas of the substructure. This provides sufficient room for the impression material. Reline, or rebase as usual, treating the cast of the bar as discussed above.

Metal Clips for Retention

If a metal rider is preferred, it should be incorporated into the prosthesis when it is initially fabricated. Instead of using the modeling rider, substitute the metal rider (Fig. 16-43). Be careful that its retentive flanges are covered with plaster before the prosthesis is processed.

Advantages of the Hader System

The Hader bar system has some real advantages over other bar systems.

1. The plastic bar pattern is easily adapted to differences in the surface of the gingival ridge and gingival curvature.
2. The plastic bar pattern simplifies the laboratory technique by eliminating a soldering step.
3. Plastic riders give adequate retention and are easily replaced.
4. Its rotational joint action relieves stresses from the abutment teeth.

The main disadvantage of this system is its plastic rider which cannot be altered for additional retention. However, the adjustable metal riders can be used to eliminate this problem. In addition, there is no provision for developing vertical function with the overdenture.

Chapter 17

Stud Attachments

Stud Anchorage Systems

Stud anchorage systems are particularly useful as retainers for overlay prostheses. They are versatile in design and application. Stud attachments consist of a vertical male post soldered to the coping and a retentive female processed directly into the overdenture or secured later with self-curing resin (Fig. 17-1). The female's retention mechanism may simply grasp the male, and thus provide frictional retention, or it may engage a special undercut so the prosthesis "snaps" into place.

Studs are generally used on short copings, where they may be mounted on independent abutments or placed strategically along a span of splinted abutments (Figs. 17-2a and b). A wide variety of studs are available, permitting the dentist to limit and redirect the maximal loading on the mucosa and the abutments.

A stud may be resilient (and thus permit a slight vertical movement) or non-resilient. Both resilient and non-resilient studs may also offer "hinge freedom" in which the prosthesis rotates much like a bar joint.

When to Use a Stud Attachment

Stud attachments may be considered for some of the following conditions:

1. For retention, stability and support for an overlay prosthesis.
2. On individual short copings with adequate bone support.
3. On individual short copings too distant from each other for use with bars.
4. For strategic placement on a splinted span of short copings.
5. For strategic placement on splinted copings when a loss of an abutment is anticipated.
6. Where vertical space is limited.
7. For maximum esthetics, not possible with most bar systems.
8. For maximum tissue support.
9. For use with copings under the denture bases of partial dentures.
10. Personal preference.

When to Use a Resilient Stud

A resilient attachment permits the tissue to compress slightly before any load is transmitted to the abutment. It is usually preferred:

1. When there are only a few abutments.
2. When abutments have minimal bone support.
3. For tissue-tooth supported prosthesis.
4. When functioning opposite natural dentition.
5. When functioning against a non-resilient appliance (do not use opposite another resilient appliance).
6. When multi-directional (stress-broken) action is desirable.

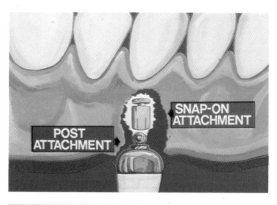

Fig. 17-1 An illustration showing the post portion of a stud attachment on a short coping. The female portion is processed in the denture base to provide retention and stability for the overlay prosthesis. A stud is an excellent choice of attachment for isolated abutments restored with a short coping.

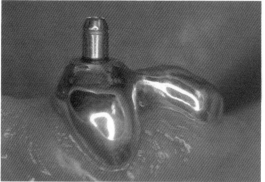

Fig. 17-2a A resilient Gerber attachment male on a short coping.

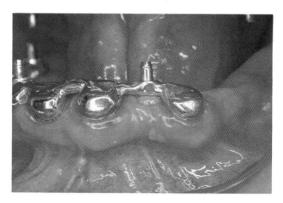

Fig. 17-2b Stud attachments positioned strategically along a span of splinted short copings. A stud is positioned in different locations in regards to abutment bone support (place the stud over abutments with the most bone support); for maximizing retention and stability by spacing studs in different planes.

Figs. 17-3a to b   The Gerber anchorage system consists of a male stud soldered to the coping and the female component processed in the denture base.

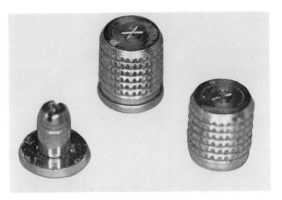

Fig. 17-3a   The resilient Gerber allows vertical movement with minimal rotational action. The attachment shown on top is the male and female assembled. The female is lower right and the male lower left.

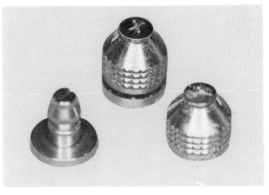

Fig. 17-3b   A non-resilient Gerber allows no vertical movement with only a slight rotational action. The assembled attachment is shown top, female lower right and male lower left.

7. When there is a minimum denture base.
8. To compensate for tissue resorption, ill-fitting prosthesis, or errors in substructure cementation.

When to Use a Non-Resilient Stud Attachment

A non-resilient attachment will not allow vertical movement (however, it may permit rotation). It is preferred

1. When no vertical movement is indicated.
2. When an all-tooth supported prosthesis is desired.
3. When a tooth-tissue supported appliance is desired.
4. With strong abutments having maximum bone support (one-half or more).
5. When functioning against a resilient prosthesis.

6. When a large, well-fitting denture base is possible.
7. When there is little interocclusal space.
8. Opposite a complete denture.

Some Stud Attachments

There is a wide variety of stud attachments from which to select:

1. Dalla Bona
2. Intrafix
3. Ancrofix
4. Gerber
5. Gmur
6. Rotherman
7. Huser
8. Schubiger
9. Ceka

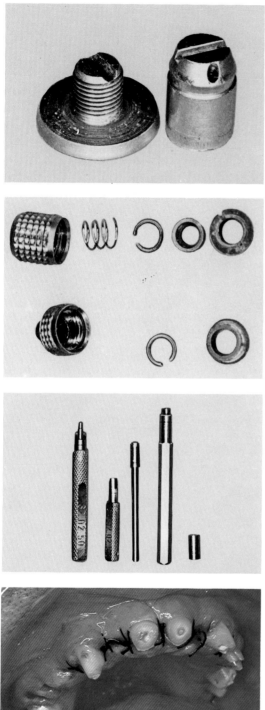

Fig. 17-4a The Gerber male consists of a threaded base (left) and a removable sleeve (right). The screw base is soldered to the coping diaphragm. The removable sleeve can be made more secure by placing a thin mix of resin inside the sleeve and then screwing it in place. A small vent hole in this sleeve allows excess resin to escape. The excess resin should be removed.

Fig. 17-4b The female component has numerous parts (top: from left to right). The internal parts of the resilient female: housing, coiled spring, C-spring, a retention sleeve, the lock screw. The non-resilient female (bottom: left to right) the female housing, a C-spring and screw cap. The latter has no copper spacer or coiled spring.

Fig. 17-4c Tools used with the Gerber anchorage system (from left to right): female screwdriver, male screwdriver, paralleling mandrel, relining tool, soldering cornal.

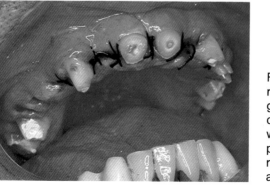

Fig. 17-5 All teeth to be retained were initially reduced to one to two millimeters above the gingiva for a favorable crown-root ratio. Exercise care not to cut the tissues and cause bleeding which will complicate endodontics (if not completed). Abutments are "rough-prepared" for a retentive adaptation of the interim overdenture after extractions and periodontal therapy.

The Gerber Attachment and its Functions

The Gerber stud system is a versatile stud attachment used routinely by the author.

It consists of a male post soldered to the coping and a retentive female secured within the denture base of the overlay prostheses.

The Gerber attachment is furnished in two different types – a resilient and non-resilient form (Figs. 17-3a and b).

The male post consists of two parts – a threaded base, which is soldered to the diaphragm of a coping, and a removable sleeve with a retentive undercut (Fig. 17-4a).

The resilient female consists of a female housing, copper shim, coil spring, a spring-retaining sleeve, C-spring, and threaded retainer. The non-resilient female has no copper shim, spring coil or spring-retaining sleeve (Fig. 17-4b).

Convenient tools are also used in the fabrication – female screwdriver, male screwdriver, paralleling mandrel, heating bar, and a soldering cornal (Fig. 17-4c).

Resilient Gerber Overdenture Treatment

A fifty-eight-year-old female had numerous upper and lower teeth. Advanced periodontal disease caused extensive bone loss. A minimum of one-third bone support remained around most of the abutment teeth. Some of the teeth had no bone support and were to be removed. The prognosis of the dentition was considered hopeless for routine restorative procedures, but good for an overdenture prosthesis. It was decided to save seven upper and eight lower teeth.

These teeth were to be reduced to create a more favorable crown-root ratio and restored with copings fitted with Gerber attachments.

Examination, Diagnosis and Treatment Planning

The precise sequence of steps for a treatment varies, and is based on a thorough oral examination, diagnosis and your answers to these questions: When will periodontics and endodontics be completed? When will the hopeless teeth be removed? Must an interim denture be provided? Will many of these procedures be combined time-wise?

This case illustrates many of the clinical and technical steps encountered with most overdenture techniques. The retained mandibular and maxillary teeth were treated periodontally and endodontically and then restored with copings fitted with Gerber attachments to support the overdentures. In this case, resilient Gerber attachments were used.

Clinical and Technical Procedures

Briefly, the clinical and technical procedures were managed in the following manner:

1. Examination, study casts, diagnosis, treatment planning.
2. Prophylaxis, soft tissue curettage, home care instructions.
3. Fabrication of interim overdenture on study casts.
4. Reduction of clinical crowns.
5. Initial endodontic therapy (may be completed).
6. Extractions.
7. Completion of periodontal therapy.
8. Insertion of interim overdentures.
9. Final endodontic therapy (if not completed).
10. Operative appointments.
11. Laboratory procedures.
12. Insertion of prosthesis.

Step-by-Step
Technique

1. As discussed in an earlier chapter, all treatments must start with a thorough oral examination. This examination should include patient history, visual examination, radiographs and periodontal probe evaluation. Accurate study casts mounted on an appropriate articulator are also helpful.
2. A thorough oral prophylaxis and home care instructions are completed before any other treatment is performed.
3. Fabricate an interim overdenture on the diagnostic casts for insertion after reduction of the clinical crowns, endodontics, extractions and periodontal surgery.
4. The abutment teeth are sectioned with a carbide fissure bur and then reduced to approximately two millimeters above the alveolar ridge (Fig. 17-5). This is easily accomplished by partially cutting through each clinical crown, first facially and then lingually. Gently snapping off the crown with a hand instrument, exert care to prevent the crown from entering the patient's airway. You may wish to use a rubber dam for this procedure.
5. Endodontic therapy is initiated or completed (if not completed earlier). Follow the endodontic techniques outlined earlier in the text (see "Endodontics," Chapter 5). In this situation, endodontics was finished later.
6. Partially prepare each abutment by removing gross undercuts. This aids in retention of the interim overdenture.
7. Extract teeth, or roots of multiple-rooted teeth which do not lend themselves to the overall long-term success of the prosthesis, or which would make home care impossible.
8. Hollow out recesses in the interim overdenture over each root. In this case, the interim overdenture will serve both as a temporary prosthesis and as a periodontal bandage (see "Interim Dentures," chapter 6).
9. Now that the teeth have been initially reduced, the hopeless dentition removed, and the interim overdenture ready for insertion, periodontal therapy can be completed in a relaxed manner with relative patient comfort (see "Periodontics," Chapter 6).
10. Insert the interim overdenture with a soft relining material (as discussed in chapter 6).
11. After several weeks of healing, complete endodontics (if not completed).
12. After tissue healing and maturation (2-3 months) complete abutment preparations for short copings with post retention.
    Reduce the roots one to two millimeters above the gingiva, conforming closely to the contour of the alveolar ridge (Fig. 17-6). Prepare the roots in a conventional manner (see "Preparations," Chapter 8). Use a chamfer or bevel margin extending into or above the free margin of the gingiva. Cut a small "cross-like" indentation on the occlusal surface of the root. This will act as an index for accurate seating of the coping and will reinforce the thin coping diaphragm.
13. Use the impression technique of your choice to produce a cast with removable dies (Fig. 17-7). When there are numerous abutments, this impression should be used for coping fabrication only. A more accurate muscle-trimmed impression of the soft tissues will be taken later for overdenture fabrication.
14. Wax the copings on these prepared dies so that the diaphragms are as thin as possible. The copings should follow the ridge contour (Fig. 17-8). The waxed patterns are sprued, invested, cast and finished.
15. Position the finished castings on the cast (lock them together with Duralay); invest and solder them to form a splinted substructure. The surface of the coping

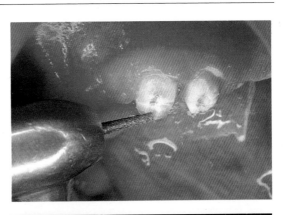

Fig. 17-6 Teeth are prepared to receive short copings after healing and maturation of the gingival tissues. Abutments are reduced one to two millimeters above the gingiva and shaped to conform to the alveolar ridge contour. The occlusal surface is indexed and the canals prepared for parallel dowel retention.

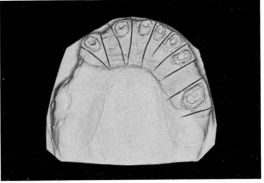

Fig. 17-7 Master cast with removable dies was produced from an impression of the prepared abutments. This working cast should be used only for the fabrication of the copings and attachment assembly. The sawing and trimming of the dies destroys its usefulness for overdenture fabrication.

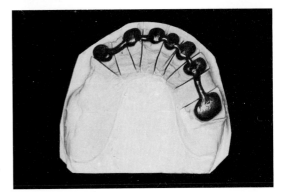

Fig. 17-8 Copings waxed on individual dies shaped to conform to the alveolar ridge. Resin dowels used as dowel patterns. Patterns should be waxed to form ideal embrasures for periodontal health.

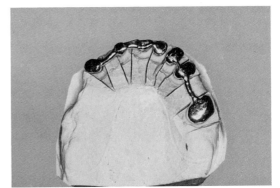

Fig. 17-9 Individual castings are positioned on their dies, connected together with Duralay, invested and soldered to form a splinted substructure. The individual copings may be fitted on the abutment teeth, locked together with Duralay in the mouth and then invested and soldered; with multiple units, the latter procedure is often preferred.

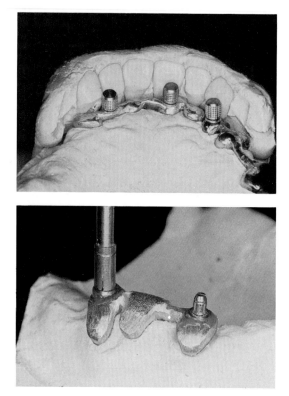

Fig. 17-10 The anterior set-up (after the casts were mounted on an appropriate articulator with intra-occlusal records) was indexed with a plaster core. The exposed lingual surfaces of the anterior teeth aid in accurate placement of the attachments.

Fig. 17-11 A male, with its sleeve loosened, is placed in the paralleling mandrel and positioned over the coping. The studs should be placed on copings supported by the strongest abutments. The studs should be placed slightly lingual to allow room for the anterior teeth, when possible.

to receive a stud, is flattened and cut with an X-ray indentation. These grooves aid in the flow of solder (Fig. 17-9).

16. Take preliminary intraocclusal relation records for a trial set-up of denture teeth. The anterior teeth are oriented with a plaster core. This helps to accurately position the male attachment on the copings (Fig. 17-10).

17. Position the male attachment on the coping. Consider the following factors when determining the position of the male posts:

   – Is there sufficient vertical space?

   – Place the posts over abutments with the most bone support.

   – Position the males slightly lingual. This provides more room for the anterior denture teeth.

   – Utilize abutments in different planes for maximum retention, stability and support.

   – The attachments must be parallel to each other and to the path of insertion of the overdenture (determined by soft tissue and bony undercuts).

18. Lock the cast (with copings) on the surveying table.

19. Loosen the male sleeves of each male slightly.

20. Place the male in the paralleling mandrel (Fig. 17-11). Find the most advantageous position for the posts taking into consideration the factors mentioned earlier. Tilt the surveying table so that the studs will be aligned to the path of insertion of the prosthesis.

21. Sticky-wax the male base to the coping (Fig. 17-12).

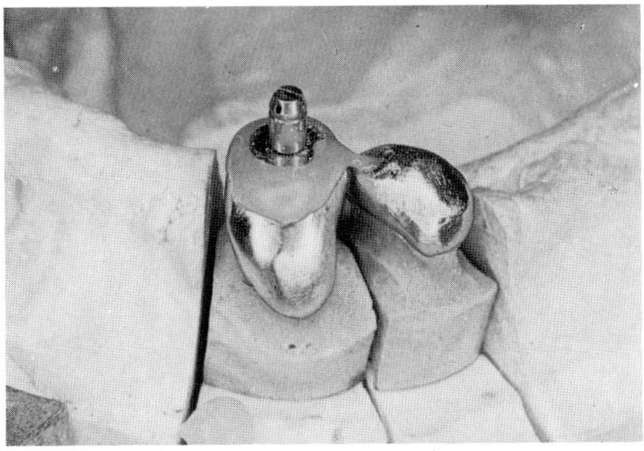

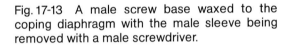

Fig. 17-12   Gerber males sticky-waxed to the coping diaphragm: first, place wax on the coping diaphragm and the base of the male, then lower the male to the coping diaphragm and apply a hot spatula to the mandrel near the male. This will sticky-wax the male base to the coping. Finally, melt additional wax up to the edge of the stud base and neighboring coping surface.

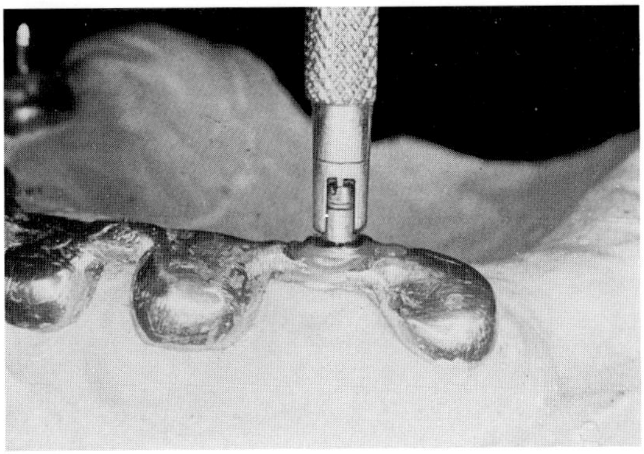

Fig. 17-13   A male screw base waxed to the coping diaphragm with the male sleeve being removed with a male screwdriver.

22. Remove the previously loosened male sleeve using the male screwdriver (Fig. 17-13). Because the sleeve is already loose, you should be able to remove it without dislodging the male from the sticky-wax (Fig. 17-14).

23. Screw the soldering cornal onto the threaded base. It acts as an extension arm for the screw to aid in soldering (Fig. 17-15).

24. Cover half of the soldering cornal and coping with soldering investment. Leave the base of the male screw and coping diaphragm exposed to receive the solder (Fig. 17-16).

25. Place the invested coping and attachment in an oven and preheat to 1400 degrees F. Remove from the oven and solder the screw base to the coping. Place the solder on the coping near the screw base so that it will be "sucked" under the

screw base. The copings are now finished and polished.

26. The substructure is placed on the abutments. The overdenture should not be fabricated on the cast used for copings fabrication. Best results are obtained if this completed substructure is placed on the abutments and a new impression taken for overdenture fabrication (Fig. 17-17).

27. Take an accurate muscle-trimmed master impression "pulling" the coping substructure, on the abutments, to form the master cast for the overdenture fabrication (Fig. 17-18).

As discussed in chapter 10, this procedure can be managed in one of two ways:

a) The substructure can be "pulled" with the impression so the substructure then becomes part of the master cast for

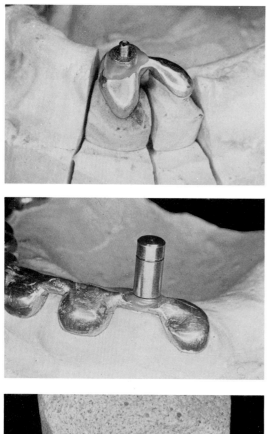

Fig. 17-14   Male stud sticky-waxed to the coping with the sleeve removed.

Fig. 17-15   A soldering cornal screwed on the screw base. It acts as an extension arm for the screw base to simplify investing and soldering procedures.

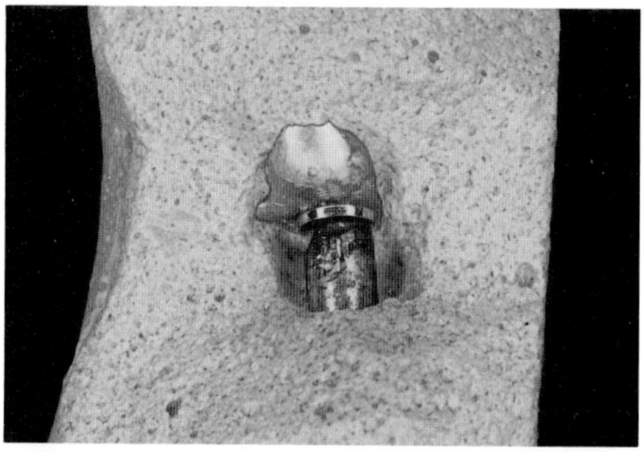

Fig. 17-16   The coping screw base soldering cornal assembly invested for soldering. The investment should cover the coping not covered by sticky-wax (accurate placement of stick-wax is a valuable aid in the investment procedure) and at least two-thirds of the soldering cornal. This will leave the bottom of the screw base and the coping diaphragm exposed for soldering.

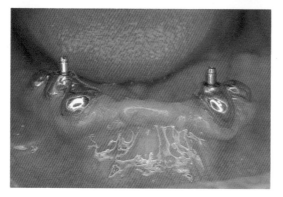

Fig. 17-17   Finished copings with the attachments assembled and soldered, positioned on the abutments.

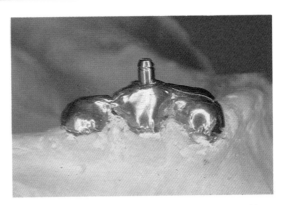

Fig. 17-18   Copings with their attachments were "pulled" with an impression to become an integral part of the master cast used for fabrication of the overlay prosthesis. The master cast used for coping fabrication is inadequate for the overlay prosthesis fabrication. The sawing, trimming and ditching of the dies destroys the accuracy of the cast for overdenture fabrication.

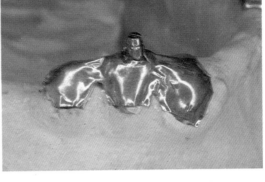

Fig. 17-19   Three to four thicknesses of X-ray foil are closely adapted to all copings for "spacing." Less space (0.5mm) is necessary for thinner and less resilient mandibular tissues than for the thicker, more resilient (0.5-1mm) maxillary tissues.

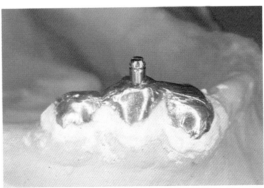

Fig. 17-20   Undercuts around all "spaced" copings are blocked out with plaster. This will prevent the denture base resin from being processed into these undercuts which would prevent insertion of the prosthesis. However, do not use excessive plaster. This produces a "dead air" space and encourages proliferation of gingival tissue.

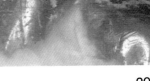

Fig. 17-21   Resilient females in place over their male studs. The females have a copper shim inside that will, when removed, provide space over the post for vertical movement of the attachment and prosthesis.

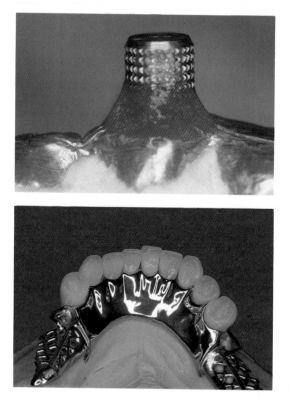

Fig. 17-22 The female-male junction is covered with auto-polymerizing resin: place Vaseline inside each female; insert the female on the male and wipe away excess vaseline; with a small brush, apply a "semi-dry" mix of resin to cover the space where the female meets the male. This resin will prevent denture-base resin from being forced into the assembled attachments. It will also improve the secure fit of the female in the denture base. Plaster, as a blocking-out medium here, is not adequate.

Fig. 17-23 A special lower framework designed with a long lingual plate festooned close to the neck of the denture teeth. A retentive mesh for retention of the resin denture base.

overdenture fabrication (as done in this situation (see Fig. 10-8).

b) The substructure can be cemented permanently on the roots and the females placed over the males. Now only the females are "pulled" with the impression. Special transfer males (as in the relining technique to be discussed later) are snapped into the females and the impression is poured with model stone. These transfer males are locked in the stone and become an integral part of the cast and ready for fabrication of the overdenture.

28. As this will be a resilient prosthesis, the substructure must be "spaced." For single copings, the aluminum spacer may be used. However, with multiple copings, other means of spacing are preferred. Thus, three to four thicknesses of X-ray foil are more easily adapted. Trim, adapt and glue the spacer over each coping to form the necessary gap between the copings and denture base (Fig. 17-19).

29. Block out all undercuts around the foil spacer and copings with plaster (Fig. 17-20).

30. Place a small amount of Vaseline inside each female then snap it (with its copper shim) onto the male (Fig. 17-21).

31. Paint a thick mix of auto-polymerizing resin at the male-female joint. This will prevent processed denture acrylic resin from being forced into the attachment during denture packing procedures (Fig. 17-22). The Vaseline placed inside the female earlier will keep out this resin.

32. Design the framework with a major connector for support and a minor con-

nector for the acrylic denture base. Fabricate and finish (Fig. 17-23).

33. Take accurate occlusal records and mount the casts on an appropriate articulator for the denture set-up (Fig. 17-24).

34. Wax, festoon, flask and process the overdenture as you would a complete denture.

35. Separate the copings' stud assembly from inside the denture. Carefully remove all spacers and excess acrylic flash. The female is retained within the denture (Fig. 17-25).

36. Use the female screwdriver to disassemble the female, remove the copper shim and reassemble. This activates the attachment making it resilient. The overdenture is ready for insertion (Fig. 17-26).

37. Cement the copings onto the roots (Fig. 17-27), and insert the overdenture. Where there are severe alveolar undercuts, trim the denture flange to improve the path of insertion.

Non-Resilient Gerber

The non-resilient Gerber attachment technique is similar to that described above but with one exception. As it is non-resilient, the overdenture and female rest on the tissues, copings and male posts in a passive position; no spacing is necessary. Therefore, do not place spacers over the copings. (Of course, the non-resilient Gerber has no copper shim spacer.)

Maintenance Consideration

Relining or Rebasing

Alveolar resorption will eventually cause the denture to rock about the abutments. This rocking will increase the rate of resorption; abutment bone support will be continually lost. Such destructive action may even cause dislodgement of the copings, breakage of attachments, or even the splitting of the abutment. The appliances should be relined or rebased to eliminate these stressful forces.

The following procedure may be used for relining or rebasing:

1. Remove the internal parts of the female with the female screwdriver (Fig. 17-28). Carefully set aside all internal parts to be reassembled later.

2. Screw the relining heating tool into the female. Heat the end of the bar in a Bunsen burner flame. The heat transfer will soften the acrylic around the female, making it easy to remove (Fig. 17-29).

3. Grind out several millimeters of the acrylic resin within the female recess. This will make additional room for the impression material and the reassembled female.

4. Place the female attachments (with their copper shims in place) over the posts in the mouth. One may wish to add a small cap of Duralay on the female. This will assure its removal within the impression. It may be necessary to grind out more resin from the recess to accommodate the additional bulk (Fig. 17-30).

5. After placing an adhesive on the tissue side of the overdenture, fill the prosthesis with an elastic impression material and take the impression using a routine complete denture relining impression technique. Have the patient close into occlusion while the impression material sets.

6. The females are retained in the impression when the overdenture is removed (Fig. 17-31). If the females are not removed, carefully reposition the females into the impression.

7. Insert the special male relining jigs (transfer males) into the females until a definite snap is felt (Figs. 17-32a and b). Transfer males are a vehicle to properly position substitute males in the same location on the cast as in the mouth.

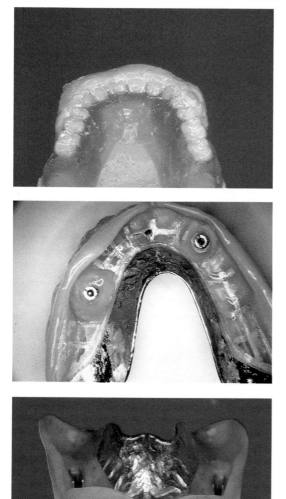

Fig. 17-24 Denture teeth set up after mounting of the casts on an appropriate articulator with accurate occlusal records: The set-up is waxed, flasked and processed as in a partial denture fabrication technique.

Fig. 17-25 Females locked inside the denture base. All excess plaster and resin are removed to expose the female. The inside components are disassembled with the female screwdriver, the spacer is removed and then reassembled.

Fig. 17-26 The overdenture is now ready for insertion. If extensive bony undercuts are present, the flanges may be reduced accordingly. The denture flange is shortened to circumvent soft tissue and bony undercuts. Denture flange extension is not necessary for retention with most attachment-retained overdentures, since retention is obtained with the attachments. The ability to festoon the denture flange often improves esthetics.

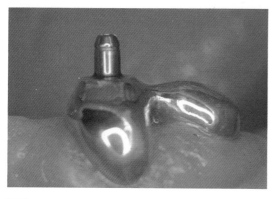

Fig. 17-27 The splinted copings with assembled attachments cemented on the abutments ready to receive the completed overdenture. The overlay prostheses should be tested for fit over the copings before cementation of the copings.

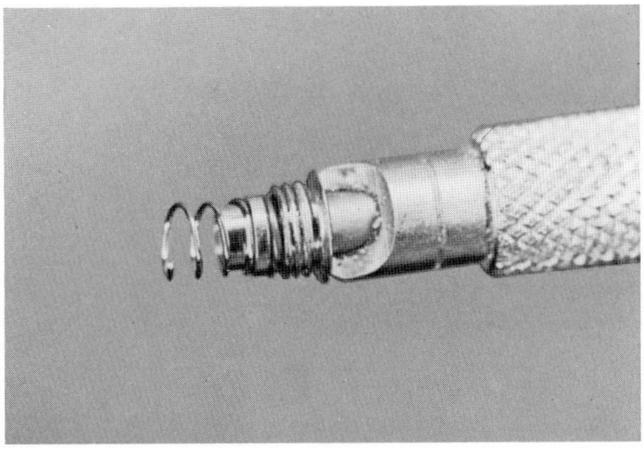

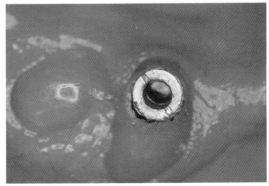

Fig. 17-28 The internal components of the female removed with the female screwdriver.

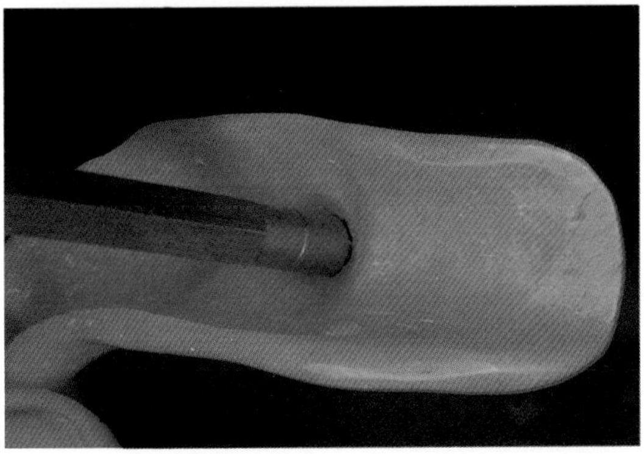

Fig. 17-29 Relining heating tool screwed into the female housing. The heating tool is heated in a Bunsen burner. Heat transferred to the female housing softens the resin, making it easy to remove. The void in the denture base is then enlarged with a number eight bur to receive the relining impression material and the female component.

Fig. 17-30 Females positioned on the male posts. The spacer is replaced in the resilient Gerber female; of course, no spacer is used with the non-resilient form. The females must have a firm snap but not too snug making them difficult to remove with the impression. A small cap of resin may be added to the top of the female to make a more secure fit of the female in the impression material. In this case the female recess inside the denture base must be enlarged to accommodate the additional bulk.

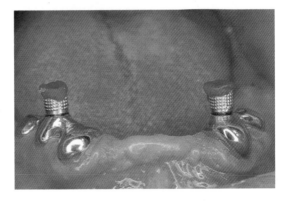

Fig. 17-31 Female retained within the impression material. If the female fits loosely, press it firmly back into position. Remove any flash of impression material inside the female.

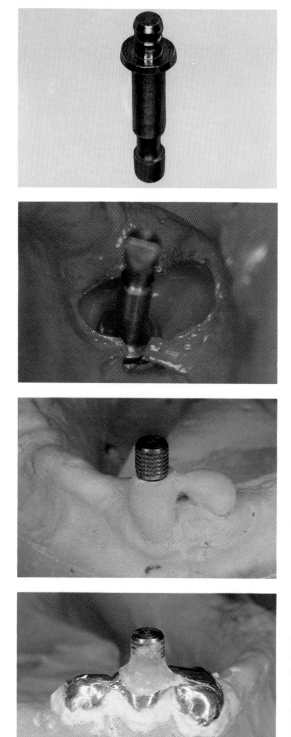

Fig. 17-32a   A special male relining jig used to produce a cast with the male stud in the same position as in the mouth.

Fig. 17-32b   Male relining jig inserted into the female. You should feel a definite snap. If the female, and male jig, is not stable in the impression, it may be necessary to secure the jig by inserting a straight pin into the impression material near or next to the jig and sticky-waxing it to the pin.

Fig. 17-33   Male relining stud extending out of the master cast with the female positioned. This cast, produced from the relining impression, is an exact reproduction of the soft tissues and coping substructure, with the male studs in the same relationship as in the mouth. This cast, used for relining the overdenture, is treated as in any complete denture relining technique procedure.

Fig. 17-34   The rebasing cast is treated as in the original overdenture fabrication procedure: spacers placed over the area of the copings; females (with spacers) snapped over the males; all undercuts are blocked out with plaster; the female-male junction is covered with self-curing resin. Then the denture teeth are repositioned from the relining jig and the overdenture rebased by any conventional complete denture rebasing technique.

8. Carefully pour model stone into the overdenture impression so as not to dislodge the transfer males.
9. The set cast, with the overdenture, is articulated to a special relining jig. The relining or rebasing procedure is similar to a conventional denture relining or rebasing technique.
10. Separate the articulator and remove the cast from the overdenture impression. The cast has the transfer males in the same location as in the mouth (Fig. 17-33).
11. The cast and attachment management is handled like the initial fabrication technique: the spacers are placed over the stone copings; females (with their copper shims) are placed on the males; all undercuts are blocked out with plaster; the denture teeth are repositioned on the cast via the relining jig, and the overdenture is fabricated by any conventional denture procedure (Fig. 17-34).
12. The overdenture is finished and ready for use.

Some Characteristics of the Gerber Attachment

In summary, the Gerber attachment is an excellent attachment system for overlay prosthetics.

Advantages of the Gerber attachment

1. It provides adequate retention, stability and support.
2. Its retention is light and easily adjustable with springs adjustable and readily replaced.
3. All of its post sleeves are interchangeable and replaceable, with the exception of the male screw base.
4. It can be used in conjunction with bars, especially when used with the Schubiger screw base.

5. It can be processed directly into the overdenture or positioned in the mouth with auto-polymerizing resin.

Disadvantages of Gerber attachment

The Gerber does, however, have a few disadvantages:

1. It is a complex attachment and maintenance problems are relatively common. The male sleeve may become loose. The internal parts of the female may dislodge when the retaining screw unthreads.
2. Its large vertical dimension makes it impractical for minimal intra-occlusal space.
3. It requires an assortment of tools for fabrication and maintenance.
4. The attachments must be parallel.
5. The Gerber permits very little rotational action, so torquing of abutment teeth will occur with alveolar resorption.

Dalla Bona Attachment

The Dalla Bona is a simple stud attachment making an excellent overdenture attachment (Figs. 17-35a and b), available in a resilient or non-resilient series. It is useful when there is minimal vertical space and where rotation, resilience and retention are desired. It consists of a single-piece male stud soldered to the coping and a single-unit female processed within the denture. It is available in two types: cylindrical and spherical (Fig. 17-36). One form even has an internal coiled spring much like the resilient Gerber. This spring helps control vertical movement. The Dalla Bona series is an excellent attachment and one used often by the author.

Cylindrical Dalla Bona

The cylindrical male post has parallel walls without an undercut. The female lamella fits snugly over the male posts, providing frictional retention. A PVC ring fits around the

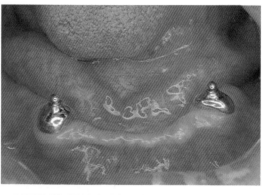

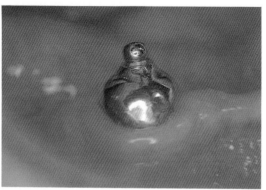

Fig. 17-35a Spherical Dalla Bona attachments on two cuspid abutments make an excellent overdenture arrangement.

Fig. 17-35b An enlarged view of the spherical Dalla Bona. Notice the excellent undercut for retention.

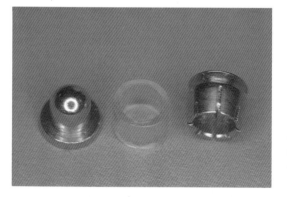

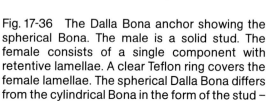

Fig. 17-36 The Dalla Bona anchor showing the spherical Bona. The male is a solid stud. The female consists of a single component with retentive lamellae. A clear Teflon ring covers the female lamellae. The spherical Dalla Bona differs from the cylindrical Bona in the form of the stud – the spherical stud is rounded in form as compared to the parallel-walled cylindrical stud.

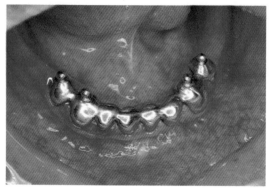

Fig. 17-37 A patient with roots restored with copings fitted with spherical Dalla Bonas.

female lamellae. This aids in fabrication, and permits the lamellae to flex. The cylindrical Dalla Bona must be parallel; therefore, the male posts must be assembled using a paralleling mandrel and surveyor.

Spherical Dalla Bona

The spherical Dalla Bona is similar to the cylindrical, but the male post is spherical. This sphere provides a retentive undercut which is engaged by the retentive lamellae of the female. If a spacer is used during fabrication, this attachment will be resilient; without the spacer, it will be non-resilient.

Advantages

The Dalla Bona attachment is a relatively trouble-free attachment that is simple to use, fabricate and maintain. It will be considered rather than the cylindrical form.
Listed below are some of the more important advantages of the Dalla Bona series:

1. Their overall length varies between 3.3 millimeters (cylindrical), to 3.7 millimeters (spherical), so it is suitable for short intraocclusal spaces.
2. It provides firm, definite retention.
3. It can be processed into the overdenture in the laboratory or mounted in the mouth using auto-polymerizing resin.
4. It is less expensive than the Gerber.
5. Parallelism of the spherical Bona is less critical than that of the cylindrical Bona.
6. The male posts can be duplicated as resin patterns. These can be mounted on coping patterns and cast as a single unit.

Disadvantages

There are some disadvantages to the Dalla Bona, however.

1. The retentive action of the female is very stiff and difficult to adjust.

2. The collar that retains the female housing in the prosthesis is too small. Therefore the female may become loose with normal adjustments and use. Often a bar must be soldered to the top of the female (in which case it must be tempered), or slots must be cut into the collar for additional retention.
3. The males must be parallel, particularly in the cylindrical form.
4. There may be some torquing and tipping of the abutment, particularly if forces are applied to the top of the cylindrical stud and if the coping is not perfectly fitted to the denture base.

Spherical Dalla Bona Treatment

Diagnosis, treatment and management using the Dalla Bona are very similar to that described for the Gerber. Differences in treatment are due to variations of this specific stud attachment.

A forty-eight-year-old female had the remaining upper natural dentition restored with a non-resilient overdenture. Lower teeth were reduced, restored with splinted copings, and fitted with spherical Dalla Bonas to retain the overdenture (Fig. 17-37).

1. The various clinical steps depend on the existing conditions. They would normally include examination, diagnosis, home care, initial preparation, endodontics, extractions, periodontics, interim overdentures, final preparations and casts with removable dies for coping fabrication.
2. The casts with the removable dies are fitted with the resin dowel pattern and the coping pattern is waxed (Figs. 17-38a and b).
3. The completed castings must be prepared to receive the stud. To improve the soldering procedure, cut a ditch in the diaphragm of the coping. This ditch aids the flow of solder under the stud base (Fig. 17-39).

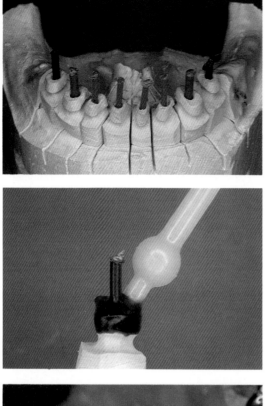

Fig. 17-38a   Cast with removable dies fitted with resin dowel patterns.

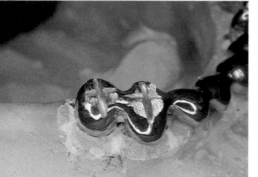

Fig. 17-38b   Wax coping patterns.

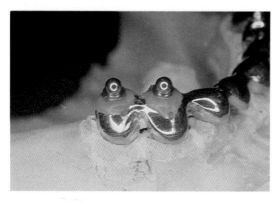

Fig. 17-39 Copings on the master cast for assembly of the spherical Dalla Bona studs. The coping diaphragms are flattened in the same plane and at right angles to the path of insertion, to receive the stud bases. The coping area to receive the stud is ditched across the diaphragm surface with an "X," or single groove. Now when the studs are soldered, solder will flow into the channels and onto the stud base making a very secure solder joint.

Fig. 17-40 Male studs are sticky-waxed on the flattened surface of the copings. Parallelism with the spherical Bona is not critical, but paralleling with a mandrel is advisable. However, the cylindrical stud must be paralleled with a mandrel and surveying table. Male studs were placed lingually to provide maximum room for set-up of the anterior teeth.

4. With the cast on a surveying table, use a paralleling mandrel to position the male studs parallel to each other. These studs should be located slightly lingual to allow room for the denture teeth. Now sticky-wax them into position. This wax should cover only the periphery of the base (Fig. 17-40).

5. Add a short strip of round wax to one side of the waxed base. This will produce flame vent holes within the investment material. This also aids the soldering procedure (Fig. 17-41).

6. Carefully invest, leaving only the top of the coping and base of the male exposed.

7. Preheat in an oven to 1400 degrees F.; this also aids the soldering technique.

8. Flame solder the male to the coping by adding solder in the prepared ditch. It will flow to the base of the male.

9. The copings with their soldered attachments are now polished and ready for assembly. Simply polish the stud lightly with a wire brush in a slow handpiece (Fig. 17-42).

10. Next position the copings on the abutments. The copings are to be pulled with the impression for the overdenture fabrication (see Fig. 17-37). With a custom tray take an accurate muscle-trimmed impression of the arch with the copings in place. As already mentioned, the original cast may be used for fabrication of the overdenture; however, the authors strongly recommend that this second muscle-trimmed impression be taken with the substructure on the abutments. The substructure was withdrawn with the impression to become part of the master cast (Fig. 17-43). (The transfer male technique is also available with this attachment, like that discussed for the Gerber attachment.)

11. If resilient Dalla Bonas are used, place the spacers over the copings before seating the females. No spacers were used since the non-resilient spherical attachment was used in this situation.

12. Place the females over the males. Position the Teflon ring to cover the female lamellae. This Teflon ring should fit flush to the base of the male. This acts as the blocking-out medium. It prevents resin from being processed inside the female and gives lamellae room to flex (Fig. 17-44).

13. Block out all coping undercuts with plaster (Fig. 17-45).

14. The casts are articulated on an appropriate articulator with accurate occlusal records for set-up of the denture teeth.

15. The overdenture, with an all-metal base is processed and finished for insertion with the female retained inside the denture base (Fig. 17-46).

16. The copings are cemented on the abutments ready for the insertion of the prosthesis (see Fig. 17-37).

Processing the Female Attachment at Chairside

Often it is necessary to insert the female into the overdenture while in the mouth. There are certain dangers associated with this procedure so care should be exercised.

1. Prepare a recess inside the overdenture to receive the female. The overdenture should rest passively on the tissues, with space around the female when inserted into the mouth.

2. Place some Vaseline into the female and snap the female over the male (Fig. 17-47). Wipe away all excess Vaseline.

3. Press the Teflon[1] ring against the male base covering the female lamellae (Fig. 17-48).

4. Place soft wax[2] under all undercuts (Fig. 17-49). This will prevent resin from locking into the coping undercuts. Severe problems can occur if this does happen.

---

[1] Teflon (registered trademark – Dupont).
[2] Jactona Corp., Dist., Philadelphia, Pe.

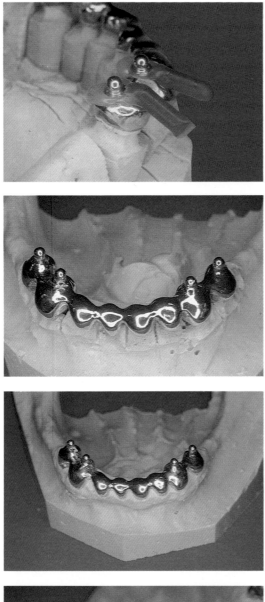

Fig. 17-41 A short length of round wax was sticky-waxed near the base of each male stud. After investing and while soldering, this wax will leave a vent for more efficient soldering.

Fig. 17-42 Dalla Bona studs soldered on the diaphragm of a short copings. The stud should be polished lightly with a steel wire brush on a slow handpiece and then polished highly with a chamois wheel and rouge.

Fig. 17-43 Coping substructure withdrawn from the abutments with an accurate muscle-trimmed impression to become an integral part of the master cast. This substructure-retained master cast is used to fabricate the overdenture. This simple procedure improves the fit, function and success of the overdenture.

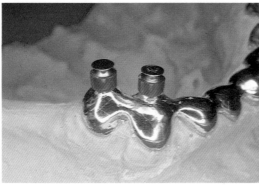

Fig. 17-44 The female component of the Dalla Bona snapped on the stud. The Teflon sleeve is positioned down firmly to the base of the stud. This will prevent processed resin from being forced into the female.

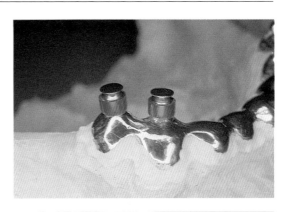

Fig. 17-45 All undercuts around the copings are blocked out with plaster. Do not use excessive plaster, otherwise there will be unnecessary space between the copings and tissue side of the denture base where gingival tissue will proliferate.

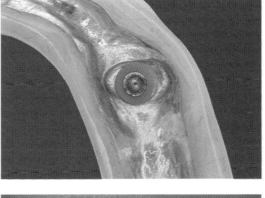

Fig. 17-46 Female Dalla Bona locked inside the denture base. The Teflon ring covering the lamellae provides sufficient resiliency for the clasping action of the lamellae.

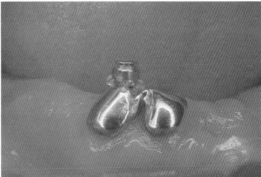

Fig. 17-47 Vaseline is placed inside the female before the female is snapped over the male. The Vaseline will prevent resin from flowing inside the female and around the male studs. All excess Vaseline is removed.

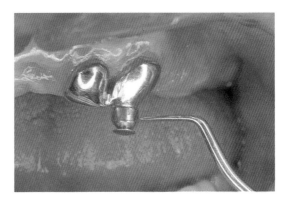

Fig. 17-48 The Teflon ring is pressed down to the male base with a blunt instrument. The lamellae and the female-male junction must be covered by the spacer. This spacer will prevent resin from flowing inside the female and around the male posts, locking them together.

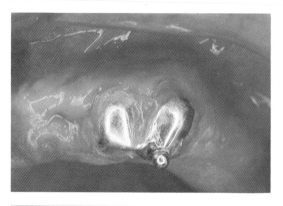

Fig. 17-49   Soft peripheral wax is placed under all coping undercuts. This will prevent resin from getting into these undercuts, locking the overdenture in place. Forceful removal could dislodge the coping crown, fracturing the abutments.

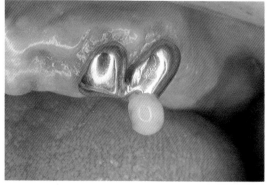

Fig. 17-50   Auto-polymerizing resin painted over the female and then into the female recess; the overdenture is then inserted and the patient advised to close lightly into occlusion until the resin sets; the overdenture is removed and all excess resin trimmed away.

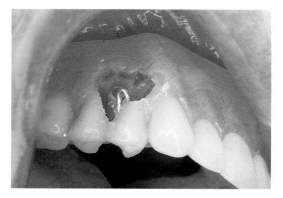

Fig. 17-51   Overdenture destroyed in an attempt to remove resin locked under coping undercuts while positioning females directly in the mouth. The coping undercuts were not blocked out with soft wax. Gingival tissue may even be traumatized if the denture base is cut away carelessly.

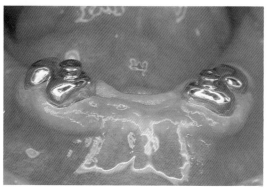

Fig. 17-52   Rotherman studs on short copings are excellent attachments to retain an overdenture.

5. Paint a thin layer of pink resin around the female (Fig. 17-50), and a minimal amount into the overdenture female recess.
6. Insert the overdenture and have the patient close into occlusion until the resin cures. Now remove the overdenture and trim away all excess resin before inserting the overdenture for use.

Use this technique with caution. For example, if the soft wax (or some other blocking-out medium) is not used, excess resin may be forced into undercuts or into the embrasure areas. This will lock the removable appliance to the cemented substructure. Using force to remove the appliance may dislodge the cemented substructure, or worse, fracture abutments. The only solution is to cut away the denture base to remove the troublesome resin (Fig. 17-51). Of course the overdenture must then be repaired.

The Rotherman Attachment

The Rotherman is another excellent stud attachment (Fig. 17-52).

The Rotherman consists of a solid stud (that is soldered to the coping) and a clasp-like female (that is mounted in the overdenture, Figs. 17-53a and b). Like many stud attachments, it is available in both resilient and non-resilient designs. The resilient form has a taller male and is supplied with special spacers.

The Rotherman is particularly applicable where intra-occlusal space is limited, as the non-resilient design has a vertical dimension of just 1.1 millimeter and the resilient just 1.7 millimeter.

The male features a definite undercut on just one side of the cylinder. A scribe line on the occlusal indicates the position of maximum undercut (Fig. 17-54). The male must be soldered to the coping so that this line (and the undercut below it) is positioned facially. This way, the female's clasp arms will reach around from lingual to engage the undercut and the bar-like retentive lug will fall in the lingual portion of the denture. There it will not interfere with the tooth set-up and will be locked in thicker resin.

The Rotherman is the easiest of all attachments to solder, for it comes with solder built into the center of the male. The technician need only position the male on the coping and then hold it in a flame until the solder flows.

Rotherman Overdenture Treatment

This condition involves a 57-year-old male patient with four remaining lower teeth. These teeth were restored with copings fitted with resilient Rothermans to retain the overlay prosthesis.

1. All clinical and laboratory steps were accomplished previously to produce a master cast with removable dies for fabrication of short copings (Fig. 17-55).
2. Place the copings on the master cast (Fig. 17-56).
3. Determine the path of overdenture insertion in regards to soft and bony undercuts.
4. Parallelism of Rotherman studs is not critical. Although it is best to parallel all attachments with a paralleling instrument, the Rotherman may be positioned closely parallel to each other in this manner: first flatten the occlusal surface of each coping to receive the male post. These flat surfaces should be in the same plane and at right angles to the path of insertion (Fig. 17-56). Cutting these flat surfaces in the same plane and at right angles to the path of insertion (on which to place the flat-surfaced studs) will automatically semi-parallel these studs (Figs. 17-57a and b).
5. Clasp the coping in soldering tweezers.
6. Place a small amount of soldering flux on the flat surface and position the stud on this surface in a lingual position. The

scribe line on the stud occlusal should point facially.

7. Hold the coping and post in a Bunsen burner until the solder flows from the middle of the stud to the coping (Fig. 17-58). Heat-treat the assembly and carefully polish so as not to destroy the undercut.

8. Assemble the copings with their studs on the cast. Again, it is always advisable to obtain a new master cast using a muscle-trimmed impression with the copings and attachments in place on the abutments. Copings with Rotherman studs are always best pulled with the impression so that they become an integral part of the cast. A stone cast of the Rotherman stud would not be strong enough to withstand the overdenture fabrication techniques (Fig. 17-59).

9. Fabricate custom occlusal registration trays to record all necessary occlusal relationship and to articulate master casts on an appropriate articulator (Fig. 17-60).

10. This is a resilient series, so adapt a spacer over the copings (Fig. 17-61a). Three to four thicknesses of X-ray foil were used instead of the aluminum spacer provided. Adapting foil is easier for multiple copings.

11. Block out all undercuts around the copings with plaster. Do not over-block-out which will produce excess space here after the prosthesis is processed (Fig. 17-61b).

12. The female clip was snapped over the post and against the foil. The clasp ends should engage the undercut at the scribe line. Pull back and up on the clasp lug until the clasp ends definitely engage the undercut (Fig. 17-61c).

13. Glue the small post spacer to the top of the stud. This will space the top of the stud. (If the non-resilient series is used, no spacing is done.) Cover the clasp arms from their tips to the clasp-retaining bar with cement or rubber base impression material, or Rubber Sep[1] (Fig. 17-61d). This is a very important procedure and must be done carefully. Otherwise acrylic resin will be packed around the post and clasp, locking them together. If you do not protect this assembly in this way, the substructure may be bent when you try to remove the overdenture after processing.

14. Duplicate the cast in a refractory material, design, fabricate and finish the framework as described in chapter 12.

15. If a trial set-up is to be made before to final fabrication, place foil over the copings and attachments before setting up the denture teeth. It can then easily be removed for verification with the patient (Fig. 17-62).

16. Finalize the set-up, then wax-up, flask, process and finish the overdenture. The substructure should be carefully removed from inside the overdenture. Do not exert exessive force lest the framework be bent. For this reason the blocking out procedure must be carried out with extreme care.

17. Remove all spacers, blocking-out material, and excess acrylic flash. Free the clasp areas, if locked in with acrylic (Fig. 17-63). This is an extremely important step. If the arms are not free to function, the appliance will "lock" on the studs and cause possible damage to the abutments if the appliance is removed with force.

18. The denture now is ready for insertion after cementation of the copings (Figs. 17-52 and 17-64).

Some Advantages of the Rotherman

The Rotherman is an excellent attachment, simple to use, and requires very little maintenance.

---

[1] APM-Sterngold, San Mateo, Calif.

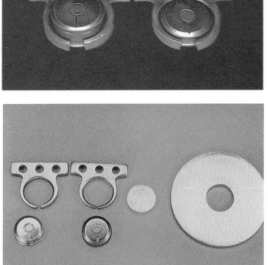

Fig. 17-53a   The Rotherman anchorage has a short, solid stud (non-resilient right, resilient left) and a double-armed clasp. The clasp has a bar for retention within the denture base. The dissimilar metal on top of the stud is solder that makes the stud self-soldering.

Fig. 17-53b   It is available as a non-resilient (left); and resilient forms (right). The resilient form is supplied with a small aluminum spacer that spaces the top of the male stud and a large aluminum spacer that is adapted to the coping diaphragm to space the copings.

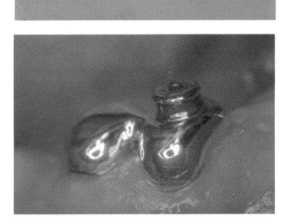

Fig. 17-54   Resilient Rotherman stud on a short coping. To provide retention when the clasp arms engage the male stud, retention of the male unit is provided by a definite undercut or "lip" located partially around its upper edge. A groove located on top of the attachment indicates the area of maximum undercut. The opposite surface of the stud has no undercut. Located through the center of the stud is a solder core which makes this unit the easiest to solder.

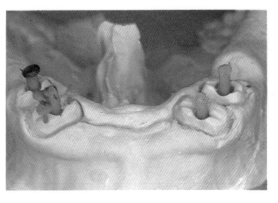

Fig. 17-55   Master cast with removable dies for fabrication of copings and attachment assembly.

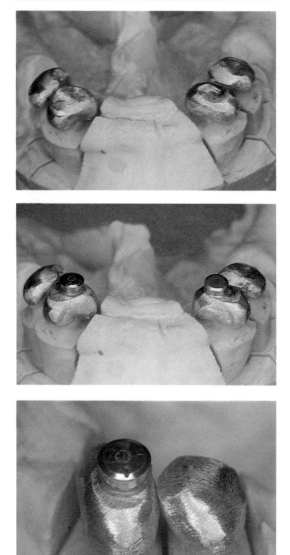

Fig. 17-56   The area of the coping diaphragm to receive the Rotherman stud is flattened in the same plane and at right angles to the path of insertion.

Fig. 17-57 a   Place a Rotherman stud on each coping (that will receive a stud) and visual-test for parallelism.

Fig. 17-57 b   You may wish to alter the flattened surface to improve the parallelism. Note that the stud is positioned with its scribed line located facially (area of maximum undercut).

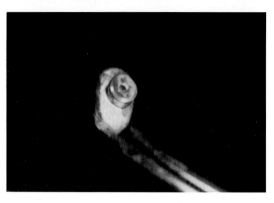

Fig. 17-58   Soldering the stud to the coping diaphragm: place a small amount of flux on each flattened area that will receive a stud; position each stud with the scribed line (area of maximum undercut) pointed facially; carefully clasp the coping with soldering tweezers; hold the coping, with its stud, over the reducing portion of a torch flame; the stud is automatically soldered to the copings as the melted solder core flows to the stud base.

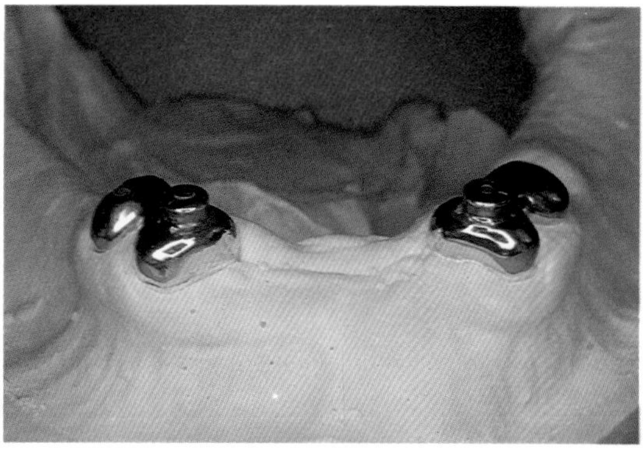

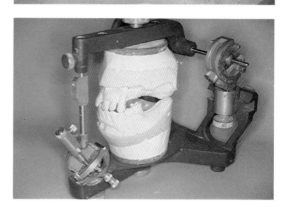

Fig. 17-59 Copings with their soldered Rotherman studs assembled on the master cast. Sawing and trimming of the dies destroys the usefulness of the original cast. Therefore, the copings were "pulled" with an impression taken for the fabrication of the overdenture to form this cast.

Fig. 17-60 Master casts mounted on an appropriate articulator with its accurate occlusal records.

1. One of its more important features is its extremely low profile.
2. It has adequate retention, which is readily adjusted, similar to the clasps of a clasp partial denture.
3. Parallelism of the males is not critical, but should be made closely parallel for best function.
4. The self-soldering center makes it the easiest to solder of all attachments.
5. The male posts do not break.
6. The female clip is well retained in the resin.
7. The male posts are easily duplicated for resin patterns.

Some Disadvantages of the Rotherman

Although this attachment has many advantages, it does have some disadvantages.

1. Chairside insertion of the female is difficult or even hazardous; therefore, the females are best processed in place in the laboratory.
2. Sufficient denture bulk must be present lingually to secure the female lug.
3. A transfer male is available for relining or rebasing, but proper orientation of this male in the impression material is difficult and error prone.
4. It is difficult to properly block out the male post and female clasp arms (step 14), so acrylic will often lock the two together in processing.

Relining or Rebasing of the Rotherman

The relining or rebasing technique for a Rotherman anchored overdenture is similar to that for other stud attachments using

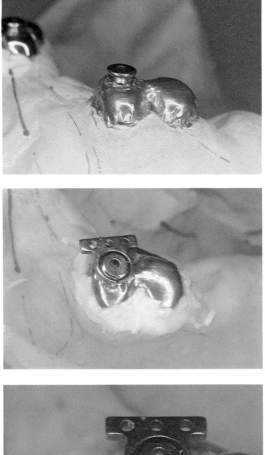

Fig. 17-61a Assembly of clasps and spacers: A coping spacer first is positioned over the stud and adapted to the coping diaphragm (four thicknesses of X-ray foil may be used).

Fig. 17-61b All undercuts around the copings are blocked out with plaster. The excess plaster should not be used.

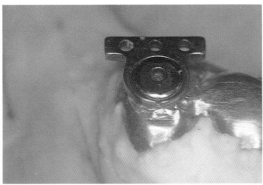

Fig. 17-61c The clasp is snapped into position. The ends of the clasp arms must line up with the scribed occlusal index to engage the stud's maximum undercut. The spacer should hold the clasp arms firmly against the stud undercut.

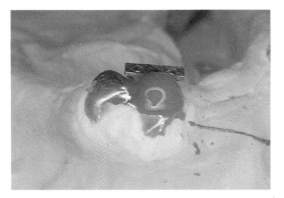

Fig. 17-61d Since this is a resilient attachment, the top of the stud must be spaced. The small spacer is glued to the top of the stud and the free clasp arms are covered with rubber impression material or a special material called Rubber Sep. This latter procedure is important and if done poorly, processed resin will lock the clasps' arms to the denture base, making them inactive. If the clasp arms are not cleared before the overdenture is inserted, there is danger of the copings being dislodged from the abutments when the overdenture is removed.

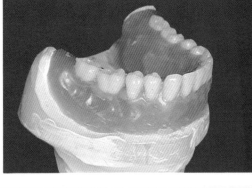

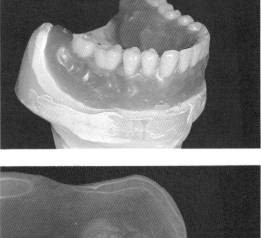

Fig. 17-62 Overdenture set-up is completed after articulation of the casts with appropriate intraocclusal records. The lingual location of the male studs provides adequate room for esthetic positioning of the anterior teeth. The clip retention bar is located lingually for anchorage into the thicker denture base.

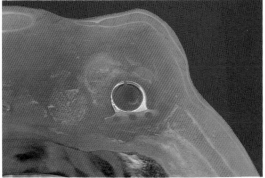

Fig. 17-63 Rotherman clips seen inside the denture base: all spacers have been removed to allow freedom for vertical movement. Any resin processed around the free clasp ends must be removed; otherwise, the resilient action of the clasps' arms will be prevented. Pass dental floss around each arm to make certain all resin has been removed.

transfer males, but with variations in technique.

1. Remove the female clip from the overdenture. Also remove additional resin to make room for impression material.
2. Adhesive the denture base and take an impression in the overdenture with an elastic impression material.
3. Insert the transfer male post into the post impression. Use the imprint of the scribed line on top of the stud to orient the transfer rebasing male in place. If the line cannot be seen, carefully position the post so that its undercut engages the impression undercut.
4. Often it is difficult to stabilize the transfer mandrel within the impression. Therefore, insert a straight pin through the impression material on either side of the male mandrel. Then sticky-wax it to the pins.

5. Using a small brush, place a thin mix of stone around the male post, the pins and neighboring ridge areas, but do not vibrate. Let this stone harden slightly. Then pour the remainder of the impression. A cast is produced with metal transfer males as part of the master cast similar to that in the mouth.
6. Articulate the overdenture with its cast in the relining jig as described earlier. The teeth are indexed in the upper member of the jig.
7. From this point, the rebasing procedure is the same as the original fabrication. (The copings are spaced, the females are positioned, the undercuts are blocked out with plaster, the post is spaced and the clasp arms covered, etc.)
8. Reposition the teeth using the plaster index. Then wax the denture and finish as in to any rebasing technique.

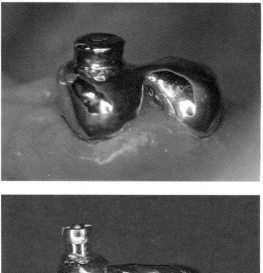

Fig. 17-64 The copings are cemented on the abutments to receive the overdenture. Allow adequate time for sufficient hardening of the cement before inserting the prosthesis. Otherwise the clasping action of the clip will dislodge the "freshly" cemented copings.

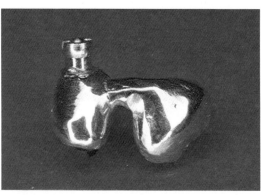

Fig. 17-65a An Ancrofix stud on a single coping.

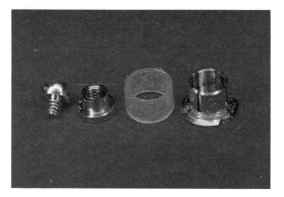

Fig. 17-65b It consists of four parts; a male stud consisting of two parts, a threaded base and a threaded retention stud; a female with a Teflon sleeve. The overall size is extremely small (3.2 mm). This screw base is common to the Introfix and therefore interchangeable.

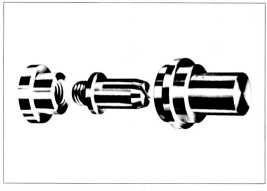

Fig. 17-66 A line drawing of the Introfix that is interchangeable with the Ancrofix. It consists of three parts: a threaded base for soldering to the coping, a root cap (a threaded, split retentive stud that screws on the male base), and the female housing.

As previously mentioned, it is often difficult to properly position the transfer males. Therefore, the authors frequently use an alternate rebasing technique that eliminates the need for transfer males:

1. After the females have been removed and the impression taken, spray the post impression with a thin layer of silicone.
2. Paint Duralay into the void left by the male post and coping. Before the Duralay sets, bend a straight pin and embed it into the material. Then pour the impression. This will produce a stone cast with Duralay males.
3. Process and finish the overdenture as described above. Then carefully examine the tissue side of the prosthesis around the attachment. If any Duralay remains, remove it with a bur.

Do not attempt to replace broken females or position them directly in the mouth with self-curing resin. Females should be replaced in a relining or rebasing procedure.

Miscellaneous Stud Attachments

There are a great number of stud attachments available, far too many to discuss each in detail. Most can be grouped with one of the systems already described. However, there are other attachments that should be mentioned.

Ancrofix Attachment

The Ancrofix is similar to the spherical Dalla Bona with a rounded male post providing the undercut for retention (Figs. 17-65a and b). Of course, the female is processed within the overdenture. This attachment consists of a male base which is soldered to the coping diaphragm, a removable sleeve knob that provides the undercut; the female has adjustable lamellae that engage the male undercut for retention. A Teflon ring covers the female lamellae similar to the Dalla Bona. This attachment is 3.2 millimeters in height and can be used in most instances a rotational action is desirable. It can be made resilient by removing the small knob located on top of the male stud and by spacing the copings.

The male sleeve can also be interchanged with the solid fixation Introfix male attachments. Thus, this attachment is indicated when a solid fixation Intrafix prosthesis must be modified to the stress-broken Ancrofix.

Introfix and Gmur Attachments

Frequently a more rigid attachment is required, particularly as support and retention for removable bridgework or overlay partial dentures, as well as for all-tooth supported overdentures. Such rigid attachments, of course, are not used if the tissue is to assume much of the load.

The Introfix and Gmur attachments satisfy these requirements.

1. The Introfix (Fig. 17-66): This attachment has a slotted, cylindrical male post that is engaged by the female for frictional retention. It consists of (1) a male base (similar to the Ancrofix base); (2) a slotted, removable stud section that screws into the male base (this latter component is split for adjustment of retention); (3) a female that fits over the male. It is available in two different sizes – 4.7 millimeters and 6 millimeters in length. Its use is indicated for retaining and supporting fixed removable bridgework, overlay partial dentures, or an all-tooth supported overdenture. Because the male post is interchangeable with that of the Ancrofix, an all-tooth supported Introfix prosthesis can be connected to a resilient, stress-broken Ancrofix overdenture.

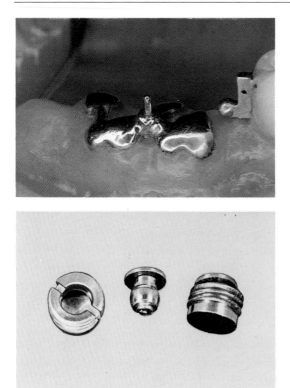

Fig. 17-67   The Gmur stud anchorage consists of two parts: a solid cylindrical rod-like stud and a retentive housing. Its use in overdenture prosthetics is limited but more useful for support under an overlay partial denture.

Fig. 17-68   The Bona-Puffer anchor is a resilient stud with a "spring-loaded" female. Note the flat-headed cylindrical stud. This flattened head provides a flattened surface to support the spring. The female has eight retentive lamellae that are more easily adjusted than the four lamellae of the Dalla Bona female.

2. The Gmur Attachment (Fig. 17-67), also is a rigid fixation stud which is indicated for supporting and retaining fixed-removable bridgework or overlay partial dentures.

The male is a solid one-piece cylindrical rod. The female contains a split sleeve that slides over the male post for adjustable frictional retention.

Bona-Puffer Stud

The Bona-Puffer anchor is similar to the resilient spherical Bona, but with some modification (Fig. 17-68). It also consists of a solid cylindrical male slightly flat on top. The "spring-loaded" female that snaps over the male has eight retentive lamellae, compared to the four on the spherical Dalla-Bona female. These thinner lamellae make it easier to adjust the retention. This is a de-

finite advantage. There is also a Teflon sleeve surrounding the lamellae.

This stud attachment has a coil spring inside the female with a vertical translation of approximately 0.8 millimeter. This translation is too large for the limited compressibility of most supporting tissues. To compensate for this vertical movement, the copings should be spaced only 0.5 millimeter, thus limiting its action.

This attachment can be used when vertical and rotational movement of the prosthesis is a desirable feature. But due to its large vertical height, more than 5 millimeters, its use is limited by the available vertical space.

The number of stud attachments available is too numerous to discuss in this text. Only those overdenture attachments commonly used were selected for discussion. This should not be taken to mean that other attachments would not be satisfactory in similar situations.

Chapter 18

Auxiliary Attachments

In addition to bars and studs, other attachment systems are applicable for overdenture prostheses. These auxiliary attachments may be in the form of screws or spring-loaded plunger attachments.

Screws

Screw Attachments

A screw attachment generally consists of a metal sleeve waxed into the pattern to become an integral part of the cast primary coping, and a screw which passes through the overlying secondary member – such as a crown or bar – to engage the threaded sleeve. A simple screw system such as the Hruska, locks two units firmly together (Fig. 18-1). It has a very limited use in overdenture prosthetics. It is more ideally used in fixed-removable bridgework. In situations where a screw may be used, often a simpler solution can be found.

Schubiger Screw Attachment

An excellent screw attachment often used in overdenture technique is the Schubiger. This attachment is a very versatile screw-type system, used with Gerber and bar combinations (Fig. 18-2).
The Schubiger attachment system consists of a threaded stud base, a sleeve that fits over the threaded stud and an internal threaded screw that screws over the stud base, locking the sleeve into position (Fig. 18-3).
Its versatility is due to the fact that its screw base is common to the Gerber screw base; it is therefore completely interchangeable. Thus, a Schubiger screw stud and bar attachment assembly overdenture can be modified to a Gerber attachment prosthesis. This attachment is indicated when doweled copings are to be splinted with a bar but the abutments are too divergent for a common path of coping insertion. This situation is easily solved with the Schubiger screw assembly. For example, the Schubiger male base is soldered to the copings and a bar attachment is soldered to the removable Schubiger sleeve. Now, the bar/sleeve unit is removed. The separate doweled copings are cemented on the divergent abutments. Then the bar sleeve unit is locked to the screw base, making the copings and bar a fixed unit (Fig. 18-2).
This attachment is considered when copings splinted with a bar may need to be removed at a later time. This removable feature is desirable when the prognosis of some of the abutments is questionable. Later, when a weak abutment is lost, the bar can be removed. The prosthesis is then modified to a Gerber overdenture.

The Schubiger Technique

This attachment would be used in the following manner after the patient was treated to produce a cast with removable dies (as in

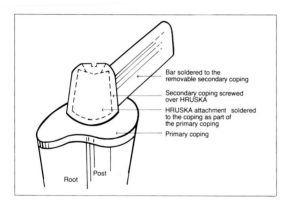

Bar soldered to the
removable secondary coping

Secondary coping screwed
over HRUSKA

HRUSKA attachment soldered
to the coping as part of
the primary coping

Primary coping

Root

Post

Fig. 18-1 The Hruska screw anchorage consists of two parts: a metal sleeve that becomes an integral part of the coping, and a screw that engages and locks a secondary member to the coping. It has limited application.

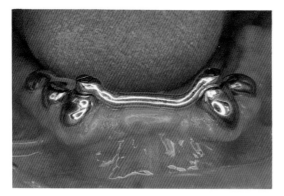

Fig. 18-2 Abutments splinted with a Schubiger bar assembly locked to a screw base soldered on the coping. The Schubiger is an excellent attachment to splint copings when the abutments have divergent paths of insertion. The screw base is soldered to the copings is common with the Gerber screw base. Therefore, the arrangement shown here can be modified to a Gerber system.

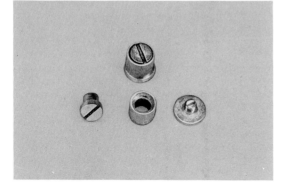

Fig. 18-3 The Schubiger attachment: top, Schubiger assembled; bottom, right to left, screw base (to be soldered to the coping); removable sleeve (to be soldered to the ends of the bars); and a retaining screw (to lock the components together).

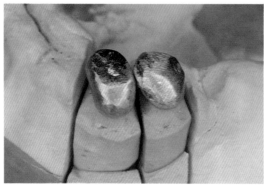

Fig. 18-4 Master cast with dowel-retained copings prepared to receive the Schubiger attachment. The coping to receive the attachment was flattened.

other overdenture treatment and attachments).

1. Doweled short copings are fabricated on the trimmed dies (Fig. 18-4).
2. The Schubiger attachment is positioned on each coping (parallel to each other using a paralleling mandrel) similar to that discussed for the Gerber attachment (Fig. 18-5a).
3. Each screw base stud is sticky-waxed to the coping diaphragm (Fig. 18-5b).
4. The screw and sleeve are removed. The threaded male base is ready to be invested and soldered to the coping diaphragm (Fig. 18-5c). A Gerber soldering cornal is screwed on the screw base to aid soldering.
5. The Schubiger posts are reassembled and the copings are positioned on the cast (Fig. 18-6a).
6. A bar is cut to length to fit between the Schubiger sleeves (Fig. 18-6b).
7. The bar is locked to the sleeves with Duralay or sticky-wax, and then removed for soldering.
8. The assembled sleeves and bar are invested for soldering. Be careful to see that sufficient investment material is introduced inside the sleeve.
9. The soldered sleeves and the bar unit are screwed over the threaded studs, transforming the single copings to a bar-splinted substructure (Fig. 18-6c).
10. A bar can be customized with a round sprue wax (Figs. 18-7a and b). Clinically and technically, treatment is similar to any bar prosthesis with clips to produce a bar-retained overdenture.
11. The copings are cemented on the abutments individually, and then splinted by screwing the sleeve/bar assembly into place over the threaded studs. This should be done while the cement is still soft. Then it will act as a splinted bar attachment system (Fig. 18-2).
12. If an abutment is lost, the treatment can easily be transformed into a Gerber system simply by unscrewing and removing the bar assembly (Figs. 18-8a to e). The screw bases retained on the copings are then fitted with male Gerber sleeves. Now female Gerbers are locked within the denture base directly in the mouth or during a rebasing procedure by using Gerber transfer males as in the technique described earlier.

Plunger-Type Attachments

Auxiliary retention for an overlay prosthesis is often desirable and it may be added to various coping or bar systems. Plunger-type units such as the Ipsoclip, Presso-matic and IC attachments can add additional retention (Fig. 18-9).

These attachments have a plunger that engages a small round depression in a coping wall or in the side of a bar (Figs. 18-10a and b). The IC and Ipsoclip systems have spring-loaded plungers, the IC being the simpler in construction. The plunger of the Presso-matic unit has a rubber cartridge which maintains the pressure on the plunger.

Ipsoclip and Presso-matic Attachments

The Ipsoclip consists of a metal plunger, a coil spring, a housing, and a retaining screw. It is available in two forms – a back-end loading and a front-end loading modification for servicing of this attachment (Fig. 18-11).

The Ipsoclip (and Presso-matic) is available in regular and high-fusing metal for soldering, or for direct-casting technique with high-fusing metal to receive porcelain.

Since the Presso-matic attachment is used similar to the Ipsoclip attachment, only the Ipsoclip system will be discussed.

The Ipsoclip can be used to increase the retention of a secondary metal coping over a

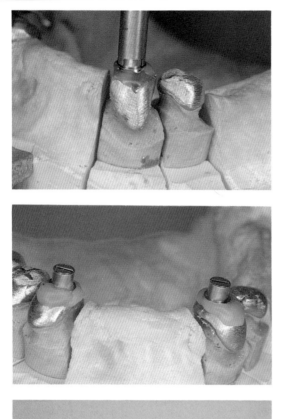

Fig. 18-5a   The assembled Schubiger unit, in a paralleling mandrel, is sticky-waxed to the diaphragm of a previously fabricated short coping. Parallelism of this attachment is critical when more than one attachment is used, especially when future modification to a Gerber-retained overdenture is expected. If a single attachment is used where one end of a bar is soldered directly to the opposite coping, the Schubiger is parallel to the path of insertion of the opposite coping and its soldered bar joint.

Fig. 18-5b   The Schubiger attachments sticky-waxed to the copings.

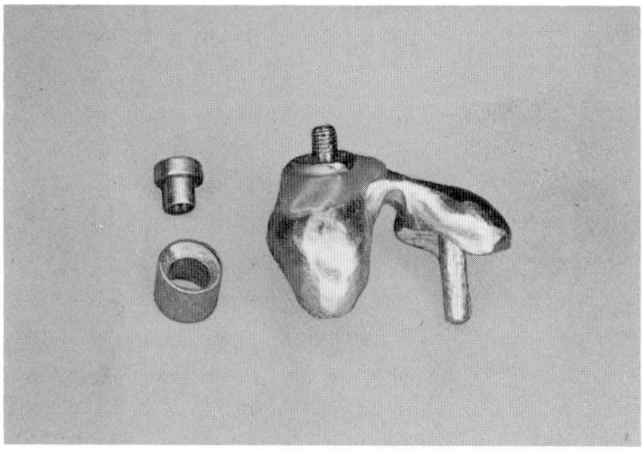

Fig. 18-5c   Copings with the screw base ready for investing and soldering. The retaining unit was unscrewed and the sleeves removed, leaving the screw base sticky-waxed to the coping diaphragm. A Gerber soldering cornal can be screwed on the male base to aid in the soldering technique.

primary coping, to improve the retention with a flat bar assembly, or to incorporate such attachments into the overlay portion of a telescopic prosthesis.

When the Ipsoclip is incorporated into the secondary coping casting, the back-loading unit is recommended (Figs. 18-12a and b). If the attachment is to be incorporated into the primary coping – into the bar rider – or inside a resin secondary coping – use the front-loading unit.

When the housing is cast directly into the metal secondary coping, it would be fabricated in this manner:

1. The primary coping is fabricated and positioned on the master cast. This coping must have a flat surface with a round

Figs. 18-6a to c   Technique for connecting the bar to the Schubiger sleeves.

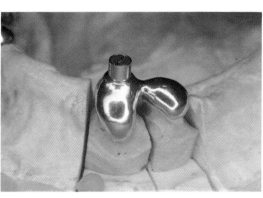

Fig. 18-6a   The copings with the assembled Schubiger are positioned on the cast.

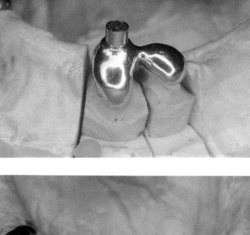

Fig. 18-6b   A bar is cut to fit near the Schubiger sleeve, in light contact with the alveolar ridge, and sticky-waxed to the sleeves.

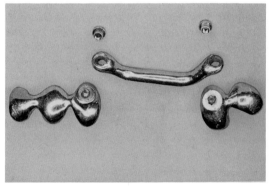

Fig. 18-6c   The sleeve/bar assembly is invested. The sleeves are soldered to the bar, polished and ready for assembly.

depression which will be engaged by the plunger. If this flat surface on the primary coping is located interproximally, then the front-loading unit is used. When lingually, then the back-loading unit is used.

2. A pattern is waxed over the primary coping to form a porcelain-to-metal substructure pattern.

3. The housing of the back-serviced Ipsoclip is waxed into a thick part of the pattern opposite the flat surface of the primary coping.

4. After its internal parts have been removed, the housing is cast with the pattern.

5. The internal parts of the attachment are reassembled after porcelain fabrication.

233

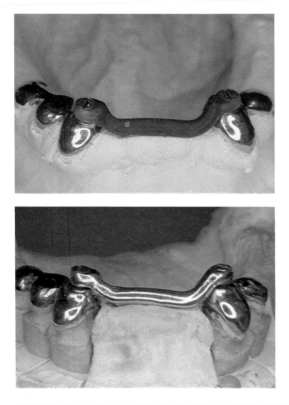

Fig. 18-7 a   A round bar pattern formed with a number ten gauge round sprue wax. The pattern was waxed directly to the sleeves with sticky-wax. The bar was cast directly to the sleeves rather than soldered.

Fig. 18-7 b   The round bar and sleeve assembly formed by the round wax sprue pattern.

6. A small round depression must be made in the primary coping to receive the plunger: the flattened surface of the primary coping (which is to receive the plunger) is air-brushed with a fine abrasive. This gives this surface a satin-like appearance; the secondary coping is inserted and removed repeatedly. This will "rub" a mark on the primary coping where the small depression is to be drilled. This depression is made at the end of the "rubbed" mark; using a number four bur drill this small depression 0.5 to 1 millimeter deep.

7. Often it is necessary to make a notch in the primary coping above the hole, or where the plunger strikes first. This helps to guide or force the plunger back into its housing until it enters and engages the prepared depression. This minimizes wear and possible damage to the plunger.

8. The overlay prosthesis is then fabricated and made ready for use. The plunger is ready to engage the prepared depression to provide added retention for the removable prosthesis (Fig. 18-12b).

A soldering technique may also be used, rather than a casting technique. When the female housing is soldered into a prepared recess in the metal secondary casting, use a high-fusing solder before porcelain fabrication, or a lower fusing solder if porcelain has not been processed on the casting.

IC Attachment

The IC attachment is another plunger-type particularly useful with resin secondary copings. The action and function of this self-contained unit is similar to that of the Ipso-

Figs. 18-8a to e   The Schubiger screw base is common to the Gerber attachment and can be changed to a Gerber system.

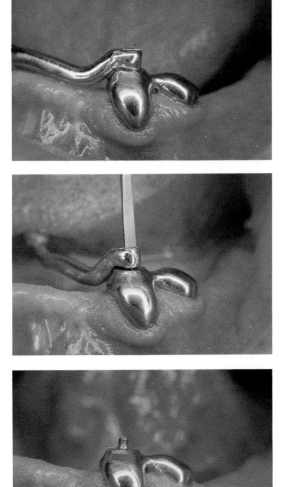

Fig. 18-8a   Schubiger bar assembly locked to the screw base soldered on the coping.

Fig. 18-8b   The Schubiger bar assembly is removed from its screw base by unscrewing the screw cap.

Fig. 18-8c   This will expose the screw base common to the Gerber attachment.

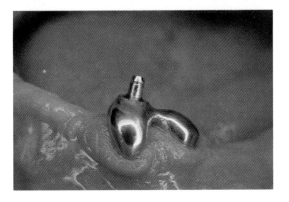

Fig. 18-8d   A Gerber male sleeve is screwed on the screw base.

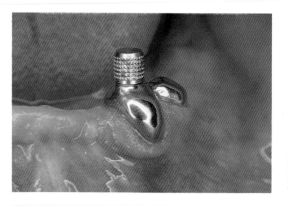

Fig. 18-8e   A female Gerber is snapped on the male and then processed directly in the overdenture in the mouth.

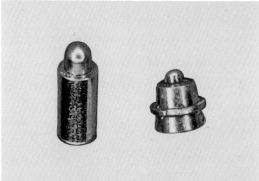

Fig. 18-9   Plunger-type auxiliary attachments (such as the IC, left, and the Ipsoclip, right) provide excellent retention when used with coping or bar-types of overdentures.

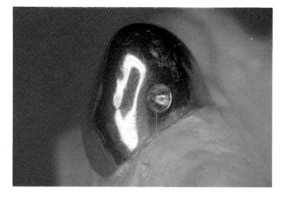

Fig. 18-10a   Coping with a round depression which is engaged by the plunger for additional retention.

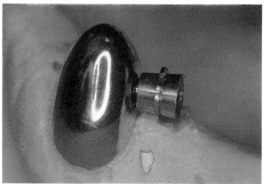

Fig. 18-10b   An Ipsoclip with its plunger engaging the round coping depression. This attachment is processed in the resin denture base with its plunger free to engage the round depression.

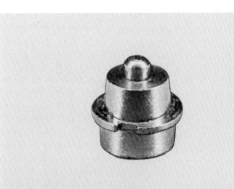

Fig. 18-11 There are two different forms of the Ipsoclip: back-end and front-end loading. The attachment can be disassembled by unscrewing the front or the back. The back-end loading form is shown here.

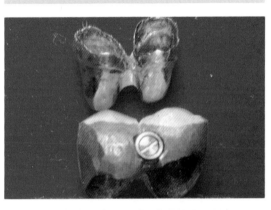

Fig. 18-12a Ipsoclip positioned in the lingual surface of a secondary coping to fit over the primary coping. This attachment is soldered in place. It can be serviced by unscrewing its back-end.

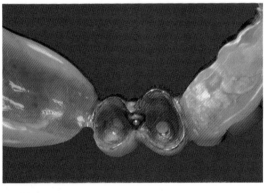

Fig. 18-12b An overdenture with porcelain-to-metal secondary coping with an Ipsoclip. Notice the small plunger inside the coping that will engage a small depression in the primary coping.

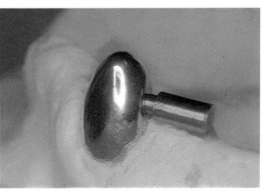

Fig. 18-13 IC attachment engaging the depression of a coping to provide retention for the overdenture. It can be held in place with sticky-wax before it is soldered more securely later.

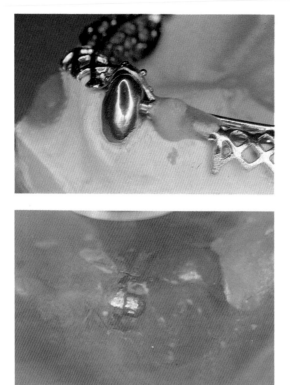

Fig. 18-14 IC attachment securely fastened to the framework with tissue-colored resin. When the overdenture is fabricated, the attachment will not be dislodged. Processed resin will not be forced around the plunger, and since the plaster will be eliminated, the plunger is free to act. Plaster is carefully placed around the plunger only.

Fig. 18-15 The fabricated overdenture with the IC attachment processed within the denture base. Notice the plunger extending out of the resin secondary coping.

clip. It is processed within the denture base of the prosthesis in this manner:

1. Drill a small round depression into the flat proximal surface of a coping (previously fabricated) to receive the plunger.
2. Insert the plunger of the attachment while holding the attachment in a horizontal position and, at right angles to the flat surface, sticky-wax the plunger into the depression. This will maintain the unit in position (Fig. 18-13). Cover only the plunger with plaster.
3. Paint tissue-colored resin around the sleeve of the attachment and lock the attachment to the framework. The plaster that covers the plunger will prevent resin from entering the attachment which would render it useless (Fig. 18-14).

4. Now the overlay prosthesis can be fabricated without fear of dislodging the attachment from its position.
5. The fabricated IC attachment telescopic overdenture is now ready for use. The exposed plunger will engage the coping depression when the overdenture is inserted (Fig. 18-15).

An IC attachment is an excellent attachment for increasing the retention of a telescopic overdenture. Often, an existing telescopic overdenture's retention can be improved by adding the IC attachment during a rebasing technique. But first, prepare a depression into the side of the coping, before taking the relining impression. Then the IC attachment can be incorporated within the existing overdenture during rebasing or relining procedures.

Chapter 19

Overdenture Maintenance and Oral Health

All too often, after a patient has had a successful dental treatment, he expects the treatment to be permanent. He assumes nothing is required on his part to maintain the health of his mouth and the fine dentistry he had just received. Nothing could be further from the truth. Such patients have to be made aware that man-made things such as automobiles, appliances and even good dentistry will not last forever. They wear out and they need constant care and maintenance to function satisfactorily for the longest period of time.

The basic reasons for the success or failure of overdenture treatment are really no different than for other dental therapy. Of course, the degree of success or failure may be to factors other than the treatment itself. Failures or problems associated with this specialized form of treatment vary. Recurrence of dental decay and periodontal disease is a serious consideration. Loss or breakage of attachment components, breakage of the overlay prosthesis, poor retention and stability, inferior esthetics, proliferation of gingival tissues around the attachments (particularly bars), copings coming loose from abutments, and even loss of abutments may be expected. These are some of the things that may be experienced with overdenture prostheses. Fortunately, most of these problems can be prevented by more thorough pre-planning. Although ways to eliminate some of these specific problems have been thoroughly discussed throughout this text,

others must be described and reviewed at this time.

There is no substitute for a thorough oral examination, including articulated study casts, radiographs, and a complete periodontal evaluation. Only when this is done can an intelligent diagnosis and reasonable treatment plan be initiated. To do otherwise is an invitation to failure, to less than ideal esthetics, to an ill-fitting appliance, or even to inadequate retention.

Overdenture Instructions

After completion of treatment, failure to instruct the patient in the proper care, use and maintenance of the removable appliance will increase the chances of breakage of the prosthesis or attachment, or even failure of the entire treatment.

For a patient to be effective in the care and use of his prosthesis, he must have a thorough understanding of the action of the attachments, if any, and the limitations of any substitute for the natural dentition.

The path of insertion of some attachment prosthesis is critical, when there are soft tissues and bony undercuts. Some attachments may or may not have a very exacting path of insertion. When selecting a particular attachment and designing the removable prosthesis, the patient's manual dexterity must be taken into consideration.

The patient should be instructed never to "bite" the prosthesis into position, but carefully to "feel" it into position around the ridge undercuts and over the substructure and attachments. Often breakage of attachments is due to this single procedure, particularly with the Zest attachment.

Similarly, the patient should be made to understand that the overlay prosthesis has to be removed with just as much care as during its insertion. When a prosthesis with very parallel attachments is removed, equal gentle pressure should be applied to both sides of the appliance at the same time. To apply more pressure on one side could lead to breakage, or wear of the attachments, dislodgement of the copings and even torquing and weakening of the abutment teeth. Frequently, it is very helpful to place a small indentation into the facial surface of the denture flange – or denture teeth – opposite the point where pressure should be applied. This will help the patient to locate the "pressure point" for removal.

Make the patient aware that the overlay denture will seem bulky at first, with little or no room remaining for the tongue. Assure the patient that this is only a temporary problem and that the overdenture will soon feel as though it is a natural part of the oral cavity.

There may also be a speech problem associated with this bulkiness. Tell the patient that this may be expected at first but will improve with time and practice. The patient may need to be instructed to read aloud until he becomes accustomed to the additional bulk. It may even be necessary to adjust the prosthesis, reshape the palatal area, or even reposition the anterior teeth to improve the patient's speech.

As with any new prosthesis, the patient may experience sore spots. These irritations may be due to over-extended denture flanges, misalignment of attachments, or even poor occlusion. These adjustments should be made to eliminate these sore spots.

Later, the patient may notice that the alveolar ridges are resorbing and the denture will rock about the abutments. The patient should be told previously of this pos-

sibility. Each patient should be placed on a regular recall program to determine if a relining or rebasing of the appliance is necessary. When a patient has all of his natural dentition, he may chew without concern. The patient must be made aware that an artificial replacement of the natural dentition is not as efficient as the natural dentition. Although an overdenture is more effective and comfortable for chewing than a normal complete denture, the patient should be instructed to take small bites, chew slowly and, preferably, to chew on both sides of his mouth at the same time. If more abutments are located posteriorly, the patient may even be instructed to concentrate his chewing over the stronger abutments. Chewing on the incisal edges of anterior teeth should be discouraged, since the anterior teeth will act as a long lever arm and rock the abutments. Of course, the type of occlusion developed with the prosthesis is an important consideration.

As it is important to keep a person's teeth clean, it is equally important to keep the overdenture clean. Cleanliness of the overlay prosthesis is important for successful function of the prosthesis, as well as for the action of most attachments. In addition, a clean prosthesis harbors less bacteria, which will improve the environment around the abutment teeth and reduce the incidence of decay and periodontal disease.

The patient should be taught the proper technique for brushing and cleaning the prosthesis. It should be cleaned with a denture brush over a bowl of water at least once a day, preferably in the evening. In addition, its removal and cleansing after each meal is important, if convenient. Furthermore, the internal portion of any attachments should also be brushed clean with the bristles of a toothbrush, or with a clean pipe cleaner.

If the mouth has a tendency to form calculus, calculus will also form on the overdenture. This calculus should be removed regularly. Placing the overdenture in white vinegar overnight at least once a week will soften most calculus and make it easier to remove. The patient should be informed that odors associated with the appliance are due to inefficient or inadequate cleansing.

The patient may notice, after a time, that the denture will not set firmly on the ridges as it previously did. It may even rock about the abutments. Before the prosthesis is inserted, the patient should be informed of the bone changes that occur when teeth are removed. That the overdenture never changes, but the ridges resorb and this occurs as a normal physiological process after teeth are removed. When this does occur, the overdenture must be corrected by repositioning the female attachments inside the denture and then relining the denture base over the copings, or, preferably, the prosthesis should be refitted by relining or rebasing.

Substructure and Abutment Instructions

Inadequate attention to motivating the patient in improved home care and the prevention of dental disease will result in eventual failure of the overdenture. Recurrence of dental caries and periodontitis is of major importance. If there is any reason for complete failure of overdenture treatment, it is these destructive factors. Therefore, home care instruction and the patient's meticulous care of the abutments and substructure are tremendously important.

Before treatment, most patients who are in need of such specialized treatment have a dentition and supporting structures in extensive stages of caries and periodontal disease. When these extreme conditions exist, effective home care techniques are almost impossible to perform. In fact, it often appears that the patient generally cares less about taking care of his teeth. Of course, after treatment all of these problems have been eliminated. What now remains is more easily and effectively managed. Generally, the patient now has a renewed interest in maintaining oral health. As a result, caries and periodontal disease can be prevented or managed more easily. Of course, this must be a team effort – with the dentist seen only as one member of this team, the patient being the other and most important team member. The patient must be made to understand that he has the major responsibility for disease control, since only he can clean his teeth daily – the dentist cleans the teeth only occasionally.

Therefore, all patients must be trained, not just shown, to use certain materials and techniques in disease control. There are some recommended materials you may suggest – dentifrice, toothbrush, flosses, toothpick, stimulating devices, disclosing solution and water irrigation devices, as well as special holding and threading devices for the picks, brushes or floss.

Disclosing solutions will color the plaque and help the patient to determine if he is doing a satisfactory job of plaque removal. The patient should be instructed in the proper use of this valuable plaque-disclosing aid.

The toothbrush is one of the main tools for plaque control, so the selection of a proper toothbrush is very important. Recommend a soft, multi-tufted nylon brush with bristles that have rounded ends. When used properly, the brush should be held with the bristles at about a forty-five degree angle, as shown in Figure 19-1. The bristles should be moved in short, circular strokes, using a gentle scrubbing action. The brush should be moved around the entire tooth surface, the copings and attachments. The object is to remove plaque and to stimulate the gums at the same time. A sawing motion is not used. Such a back-and-forth brushing action may even do damage to the root and supporting tissues.

Each stud or bar attachment should be brushed, in addition to the abutments and copings. Brush the facial, lingual, and occlusal surfaces (Fig. 19-2).

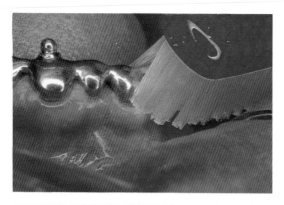

Fig. 19-1   A soft toothbrush with its bristles held at a forty-five degree angle against the gingiva, copings and bar. The brush is moved in short circular strokes and not in a back-and-forth sawing action.

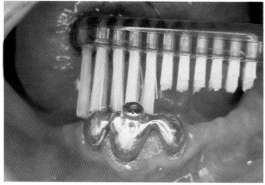

Fig. 19-2   Brushing the attachments to remove all plaque and food debris.

Often a modified toothbrush will help to reach the more difficult inaccessible lingual areas (Fig. 19-3).

Although brushing may remove most plaque, it alone will not do a thorough cleaning job between the abutments or under the bar attachments. The most valuable tool to clean these hard-to-reach areas is dental floss (Fig. 19-4). Recommend unwaxed dental floss, or a special floss called "Super Floss." This floss is much thicker, has stiff ends which act as threaders, and is an excellent interproximal plaque remover.

The patient should be instructed to wrap the floss around the side of the abutments and move it up and down to remove the plaque. He should not saw the floss back and forth, as this will damage root abutments.

Special interproximal brushes (Fig. 19-5), or toothpicks mounted in a handle for ease of manipulation, are also helpful aids for removing plaque between the crowns of teeth.

Such brushes or toothpicks are particularly useful in places where the interproximal spaces are wide enough to accommodate them. They should be inserted from one side and then through the opposite side of the interproximal spaces.

A soft balsa wood pick called "Stimudent" (Fig. 19-6), is excellent for removing plaque around the abutment roots, copings, attachments and interproximally. When placed interproximally, or around the gingiva, it stimulates the tissues, improves circulation and promotes the health of tissues.

When there are numerous splinted abutments, with close interproximal spaces, irrigating devices are very effective for removing loose food debris. The water pressure should be set low-to-medium when directing the stream of water between the crowns, around the abutments and under the bar attachments. This will remove most loose food debris; but remember, they are but one

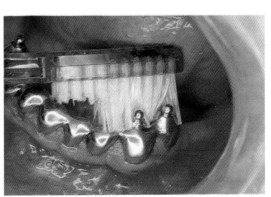

Fig. 19-3 A toothbrush trimmed for better access to the more difficult lingual areas. The bristles can be removed with a scalpel or sharp scissors.

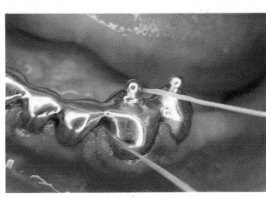

Fig. 19-4 Unwaxed floss is used to remove plaque from the interproximal surfaces of the copings. The floss is moved up and down as it is moved back and forth. It should be passed gently toward the gingival sulcus but not to injure the periodontal attachments. Wrap the floss partly around the coping to clean as much of the coping surface as possible.

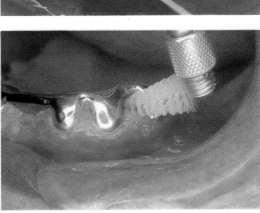

Fig. 19-5 An interproximal brush is passed through the more open interproximal areas. It is gently moved back and forth from the facial and then to the lingual direction.

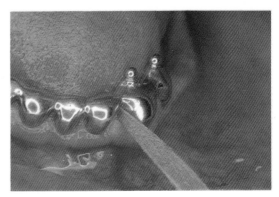

Fig. 19-6 A Stimudent, a soft wooden pick, being used to remove plaque and at the same time stimulate the gingiva. Chewing its end will soften and moisten the pick, making it more effective for removing plaque and stimulating the gingiva.

tool in oral hygiene maintenance. They will not remove plaque, however, and must be used in conjunction with toothbrushing and flossing for total plaque removal from all areas.

Shannon and *Cronin* have shown the tremendous benefits of frequent applications of a low-concentration stannous fluoride solution as a home care mouthwash program in preventing dental caries around exposed abutment roots.

They recommended the patient be given a stable, water-free 0.4 percent SnF2 gel for use at bedtime. After a thorough brushing, the gel is brushed on the abutments and the gel is swished around for thirty seconds. After the gel remains in the mouth for two minutes, the patient expectorates but does not rinse. The overdenture should be left out of the mouth and stored in a cleaning solution overnight.

The patient needs to understand that the battle to prevent dental disease through a plaque-control program has to include a sound nutritional program to be effective. Proper nutrition is the other side of the battle for dental health. The patient must be counseled on proper diet for the prevention of dental disease.

Thus, the patient has to be told that keeping his mouth healthy and free from dental disease is a team effort. Only he can really prevent dental caries and periodontal disease. You, the dentist, can only help! If dental health is important to the patient, he must take that big step forward. He must remove bacteria-laden plaque from his teeth and substructure daily and he must eat nutritional, sugarless, well-balanced meals. Only then can he enjoy the benefits of this specialized overdenture treatment and improved comfort, function, and appearance.

Bibliography

Applegate, O. C.:
> The partial denture base. J. Prosthet. Dent., 5, pp. 636-645, 1955.

Armstrong, R. L., and Boone, M. E.:
> Endodontics and the overdenture. J. Georgia Dent. Assn., Feb. 1978.

Bear, S. E.:
> Surgical correction of oral anomalies as related to dental prosthesis. Dent. Clin. N. Amer., 8, p. 337, 1964.

Boone, M. S., and Armstrong, R. L.:
> The overdenture and alveolar bone preservation, J. Maryland State Dental Association 20 (2), pp. 86-88, Aug. 1977.

Boucher, C. O.:
> The relining of complete dentures. J. Prosthet. Dent., 30, p. 521, 1973.

Boucher, C. O., Hickey, J. C., and Zarb, G. A.:
> Prosthodontic treatment for edentulous patients. St. Louis, The C. V. Mosby Co., 1975.

Brewer, A. A., and Fenton, A. H.:
> The overdenture. Dent. Clin. N. Amer., pp. 723-796, Oct. 1973.

Brewer, A. A., and Morrow, R. M.:
> Overdenture. St. Louis, The C. V. Mosby Co., 1975.

Buchman, J. M., and Menekratis, A.:
> Complete and anchored dentures. Philadelphia, J. B. Lippincott Co.

Carsten, V. F., and Cardinale, P. J.:
> The overdenture – a review, New York State Dental Association, J., 44 (8), pp. 331-334, Oct. 1978.

Christensen, F. T.:
> Relining techniques for complete dentures. J. Prosthet. Dent., 26, p. 373, 1971.

Collett, H. A.:
> Psychodynamic study of abnormal reaction to dentures. J. Amer. Dent. Assn., 51, pp. 451-546, 1955.

Crum, R. J., and Loiselle, R. J.:
> Oral preparation and proprioception; a review of the literature and its significance to prosthodontics. J. Prosthet. Dent., 28, pp. 215-230, 1972.

Dodge, C. A.:
> Prevention of complete denture problems by use of "overdentures". J. Prosthet. Dent., 30, pp. 403-411, Oct. 1923.

Dolder, E. J., and Durrer, G. T.:
> The bar-joint denture. Chicago, Quintessence Publishing Co., 1979.

Dolder, R. F.:
> The bar-joint mandibular denture. J. Prosthet. Dent., 11, pp. 689-707, 1961.

Fechtner, J. L.:
> Treatment planning. Dent. Clin. N. Amer., 22, pp. 219-230, 1978.

Federich, D. R.:
> Using hemisected teeth to support removable partial overdentures (11). Quintessence Int., 9, pp. 21-25, 1978.

Fenton, A. H.:
> Interim overdentures, J. Prosthet. Dent., 36 (1), pp. 4-12, July 1976.

Frantz, W. R.:
> The use of natural teeth in overlay dentures. J. Prosthet. Dent., 34, pp. 135-140, 1975.

Friedman, S.:
> Effective use of diagnostic data. J. Prosthet. Dent., 22, p. 111, 1969.

Frisch, J., Levin, M. P., and Bhaskar, S. N.:
> The use of tissue conditioners in periodontics. J. Periodont., 39, pp. 359-361, 1968.

Garver, P. G., Fenster, R. K., Baker, R. D., and Johnson, D. L.:
> Vital root retention; a preliminary report. J. Prosthet. Dent., 40, pp. 23-28, 1978.

Gattozzi, J. G., Okeson, J. P., Unger, J. W., and Woodward, J. D.:
> The overlay denture – what and why? J. Kentucky Dent. Assn., 27, pp. 17-20, Oct. 1975.

Gehl, D. H.:
> Overlay of tooth-supported dentures. J. State Dent. Soc., 47, pp. 362-363, 1971.

Gerber, A.:
Retentions-Zylinder und Retentions-Puffer für Brücken und Prothesen mit verdeckten Verankerungen, Cendros and Metaux, Biel, 1966.

Gilmore, S. F.:
A method of retention. J. Allied Dental Society, 9, pp. 118-122, 1913.

Glickman, I.:
Clinical periodontology, Ed. 3, Philadelphia, W. B. Saunders Co., 1964.

Goldman, B. M., and *Shannon, I. L.:*
Application of fluoride to denture surface. J. Georgia Dent. Assn., 46, pp. 17-22, 1973.

Goldman, H. M., and *Cohen, D. W.:*
Periodontal therapy, Ed. 5, St. Louis, The C. V. Mosby Co., 1973.

Guyer, S. A.:
Selectively retained vital roots for partial support of overdentures; a patient report. J. Prosthet. Dent., 33, pp. 258-263, 1975.

Helft, M., Kaufman C., and *Cardash, H. S.:*
The overdenture a concept. Israel J. Dent. Med., 27, (2), pp. 5-7, April 1978.

Isaacson, G. O.:
Telescope crown retainers for removable partial dentures. J. Prosthet. Dent., 22, p. 436, 1969.

Jaggers, J. H.:
A method of verifying parallelism of preparations for Zest anchor attachments. J. Prosthet. Dent., 39, pp. 230-231, Feb. 1978.

Johnston, J. F., Phillips, R. W., and *Dykema, R. W.:*
Modern practice in crown and bridge prosthodontics. Ed. 2, Philadelphia, W. B. Saunders Co., 1965.

Kabcenell, J. L.:
Tooth-supported complete dentures, J. Prosthet. Dent., 26, pp. 251-257, Sept. 1971.

Kalista, W. T., Jr.:
Tooth-supported complete dentures. Dent. Stud., 49, pp. 38, 58, 63, 1971.

Kay, W. D., and *Abes, M. S.:*
Exercising perception in overdenture patients. J. Prosthet. Dent., 35 (6), pp. 615-619, June 1976.

Kelly, E. K.:
The prosthodontist, the oral surgeon, and denture supporting tissues. J. Prosthet. Dent., 16, p. 464, 1966.

Kotwal, K. R.:
Outline of standards for evaluating patients for overdentures. J. Prosthet. Dent., 37 (2), pp. 141-146, Feb. 1977.

Kurth, L. E.:
Balanced occlusion. J. Prosthet. Dent., 4, pp. 150-167, 1954.

Lam, R. V.:
Effect of root implants on resorption of residual ridges. J. Prosthet. Dent., 27, p. 311, 1972.

Landa, J. S.:
Trouble shooting in complete denture prosthesis. J. Prosthet. Dent., 10, p. 3, 1960.

Loiselle, R. J., Crum, R. J., Rooney, G. I., and *Stueur, C. H.:*
The physiologic basis for overlay denture. J. Prosthet. Dent., 28, pp. 3-12, July 1972.

Lord, J. L., and *Teel, S.:*
The overdenture. Dent. Clin. N. Amer., 13, pp. 871-881, 1969.

Manly, R. S., Pfoffman, L. C., Lathrop, D. D., and *Keyser, J.:*
Oral sensory threshholds of persons with natural and artificial dentitions. J. Dent. Res., 31, pp. 305-310, 1952.

Marquardt, G. L.:
Dolder bar-joint mandibular overdenture; a technique for non-parallel abutment teeth. J. Prosthet. Dent., 36, pp. 101-111, 1976.

Mascola, R. F.:
The root retained complete denture. J. Amer. Dent. Assn., 92, pp. 586-587, 1976.

Maurer, C. R.:
Complete denture construction on alveolar process containing endodontically treated roots. J. Prosthet. Dent., 30, pp. 756-758, Nov. 1973.

McCracken, W. L.:
Differential diagnosis, fixed or removable partial dentures. J. Amer. Dent. Assn., 63, pp. 767-775, 1961.

Mensor, M. C.:
The rationale of a resilient hinge-action stress breaker. J. Prosthet. Dent., 20, p. 204, 1968.

Mensor, M. C.:
Classification and selection of attachment. J. Prosthet. Dent., 29, p. 497, 1973.

Mensor, M. C.:
Attachment stabilization of the overdenture. Quintessence Int., 4, pp. 25-28, 1976.

Mensor, M. C., Jr.:
Attachment fixation of the overdenture. J. Prosthet. Dent., 39, pp. 18-19, 1978.

Miles, A. E. W.:
"Sans teeth"; changes in oral tissues with advancing age. Proc. Roy. Soc. Med., 65, pp. 801-806, 1972.

Miller, P. A.:
Complete dentures supported by natural teeth. J. Prosthet. Dent., 8, p. 924, 1958.

Miller, P. A.:
Complete dentures supported by natural teeth. Texas Dent. J., 83, pp. 4-8, 1965.

Moffa, J. P., Razzano, M. R., and Doyle, M. J.:
Pins – a comparison of their retentive properties. J. Amer. Int. Assn., 78, pp. 529-535, 1969.

Morto, L. P.:
Telescope dentures. J. Prosthet. Dent., 29, pp. 151-156, Feb. 1973.

Morrow, R. M., Rudd, K. D., Birmingham, F. D., and Larkin, J. P.:
Immediate interim tooth-supported complete dentures. J. Prosthet. Dent., 30, pp. 695-700, 1973.

Moulton, R.:
Psychological problems associated with complete denture service. J. Amer. Dent. Assn., 33, pp. 476-485, 1946.

Nicholson, R. J., Stark, M. M., and Scott, H. E.:
Calculus and stain removal from acrylic resin dentures. J. Prosthet. Dent., 40, p. 326, 1968.

Ortman, L. F.:
Patient education and complete denture maintenance. Dent. Clin. N. Amer., 21, pp. 359-367, 1977.

Ortman, H. R.:
Factors of bone resorption of the residual ridge. J. Prosthet. Dent., 12, pp. 429-440, 1962.

Ortman, H. R.:
Complete denture occlusion. Dent. Clin. N. Amer., 21, pp. 299-320, 1977.

Pickett, H. G., Appleby, R. G., and Osborn, M. O.:
Changes in the denture-supporting tissues associated with the aging process. J. Prosthet. Dent., 27, p. 257, 1972.

Preiskel, H. W.:
Precision attachments in dentistry, Ed. 2, St. Louis, The C. V. Mosby Co., 1973.

Renner, R. P., Foerth, D., and Levey, M.:
Preventive prosthodontics – Overdenture service, N. Y. State Dental Assn., J. 43 (1), pp. 17-21, Jan. 1977.

Renner, R. P., Foerth, D., and Pessprilla, F.:
Maintenance of root integrity and periodontal health under overdentures; a pilot study. J. Gen. Dent., 26 (1), pp. 42-46, Jan-Feb. 1978.

Richard, G. F., Sarka, R. J., Arnold, R. M., and Knowles, K. I.:
Hemisected molars for additional overdenture support. J. Prosthet. Dent., 38, pp. 16-21, 1977.

Reitz, P. V., Marshall, M. G., and Levin, B.:
An overdenture survey. Preliminary report, J. Prosthet. Dent., 37 (3), pp. 246-257, March 1977.

Roberts, A. L.:
The effects of outline and form upon denture stability and retention. Dent. Clin. N. Amer., 4, pp. 293-303, 1960.

Rothenberg, L. I. A.:
Overlay dentures for the cleft palate patient. J. Prosthet. Dent., 37, pp. 327-329, 1977.

Sandoval, E., and Shannon, I. L.:
Fluoride and denture solubility. Texas Rep. Med., 27, pp. 111-116, 1969.

Schweitzer, J. M.:
Discussion of crown and sleeve retainers for removable partial dentures. J. Prosthet. Dent., 16, pp. 1086-1089, 1966.

Schweitzer, J. M., Schweitzer, R. D., and Schweitzer, J.:
The telescoped complete denture: a research report at the clinical level, J. Prosthet. Dent. 26, pp. 357-372, Oct. 1971.

Shannon, I. L., and Cronin, R. J., Jr.:
Chemical protection of tooth surfaces in patients with overdentures. In Brewer, A., and Morrow, R. (Eds.). Overdentures, St. Louis, The C. V. Mosby Co., (pp. 237-247) 1975.

Sharry, J. J.:
Complete denture prosthesis. Chapters 8 and 14. New York, McGraw-Hill Book Co., 1968.

Silverman S. I.:
The psychological consideration in denture prosthetics, J. Prosthet. Dent., 8, p. 4, 1958.

Strohaver, R. A., and Trovillion, H. M.:
Removable partial dentures. J. Prosthet. Dent., 35 (6), pp. 624-629, June 1976.

Swenson, M. G., and Terkla, L. G.:
Partial dentures. St. Louis, The C. V. Mosby Co., 1959.

Taylor, R. L., Duckmanton, N. A., and Boyks, G.:
Overlay dentures – philosophy and practice I. Aust. Dent. 21 (5), p. 429, Oct. 1976.

Thayer, H. H., and Caputo, A. A.:
Effects of overdentures upon removing oral structures. J. Prosthet. Dent., 37 (4), pp. 374-381, April 1977.

Tucker, K. M.:
Relining complete dentures with the use of a functional impression. J. Prosthet. Dent., 16, p. 1054, 1964.

Unger, J. W., Gattozzi, J. G., Woodward, J. D., and Okeson, J. P.:
The overlay denture – how. J. Kentucky Dent. Assn., 28, pp. 24-27, Jan. 1976.

Unger, J. W., Gattozzi, J. G., and Okeson, J.:
The overlay denture – then what? J. Kentucky Dent. Assn., 28, pp. 11-13, April 1976.

Warren, A. B., and Caputo, A. A.:
Load transfer to alveolar bone as influenced by abutment designs for tooth-supported dentures. J. Prosthet. Dent., 33, p. 137, 1975.

Weinberg, L. A.:
Atlas of removable partial denture prosthodontics. St. Louis, The C. V. Mosby Co., 1969.

Weine, F. S.:
Endodontic therapy. St. Louis, The C. V. Mosby Co., 1972.

Welker, W., and *Kramer, D.:*
Waxing tooth copings for overdentures. J. Prosthet. Dent., 32, pp. 668-671, 1974.

White, J. T.:
Abutment stress in overdentures. J. Prosthet. Dent., 40, pp. 17, 18, 1978.

Yahsove, I. L.:
Crown and sleeve coping retainers for removable partial prosthesis. J. Prosthet. Dent., 16, p. 1069, 1966.

Zamikoff, I. L.:
Overdentures – theory and technique, J. Amer. Dent. Assn., 86, pp. 853-857, April 1973.

Subject Index

A

Abutment(s)
bone support for — 27
clinical reduction of — 75
copings for — 36, 38
endodontic evaluation — 36, 39
examination — 75
location in occlusal plane — 45
periodontal surgery — 39, 41
preparation — 76
  long — 81, 83, 84
  medium — 77, 78
  short — 76
removable overlay prosthesis — 20
retention — 78, 84
root form — 26
selection criteria — 45
stability of — 28
Ackerman bar attachment — 142, 188, 191
Ancrofix attachment — 226, 227
Andrews bar — 141
Attachments
auxillary — 136, 142, 229, 237
  IC — 136, 139, 234, 238
  Ipsoclip — 136, 139, 141
  screws — 136, 139
bars — 136, 138, 141
  Ackerman — 142, 185
  Andrews — 141
  Ceka — 141, 185
  C. M. bar — 141, 185
  customized bars — 142, 186, 188
  Dolder — 136, 175, 185
  Hader — 136, 190, 193
  M. F. channels — 141, 185
  Octalink — 141, 185
criteria for selection — 136, 137
EM attachment selector — 136
extra-coronal — 136
  studs — 136
  Ancrofix — 145, 226

  Ceka — 142
  Dalla Bona — 136, 139, 141, 142, 213-219
  Gerber — 136, 197-213
  Gmur — 142, 227, 228
  Huser — 142
  Rotherman — 136, 219-227
  Schubiger — 142, 230-234
Attachments-Cont'd
intra-coronal — 136
  Zest — 136, 137, 153, 172
  Mini-zest — 136, 137, 167, 169
  Ginta — 136
non-resilient — 137, 138
resilient — 136, 137
Auto-polymerizing technique — 73, 74

B

Bar(s) — 136, 138, 172, 185
Ackerman — 185, 191
Ceka — 141, 185
C. M. bars — 141, 185
customized — 188
  retentive clips — 188
  Ackerman — 188
  Baker — 188
  Dolder shell — 188
  Hader — 188
Dolder — 172, 185
  impression for — 175, 176
  laboratory procedure — 177, 180
  management of — 175, 176
  retention — 175
Hader — 185, 190, 197
  advantage — 193
  disadvantage — 193
  impression for — 191, 193
  relining — 193
M. F. channels — 141, 185
Selection of — 138, 141, 185
  non-resilient — 185

Dolder bar unit   185, 175, 176
    resilient   175, 180
Dolder bar joint   175, 183
Bona-puffer attachment   228

C

Copings
    adaptation of   42
    auxiliary attachment   119
    bar attachment of   119
    basic types   45, 46
    classification   36, 37
    cementation of   43
    contour of   45, 49, 113, 115
    Cost see Fees
    design consideration   113, 115, 119
    esthetic evaluation   116
    impression for   42
    length of   36
    long   38, 46
       contour   47
       requirements   46
    medium   37, 48, 49
    Para-Post procedure for   89
    paralleling devices used   86
    preparation for   86
       CI post   86, 88, 89
       drills   86
       Para-Max parallator   86
       pins   87
       posts   86
    primary   115
    retention   116
    secondary   45
    splinted   94
    types   85
       dowel (post)   85
       non-parallel   85
       parallel   85
    vital teeth   68
    waxing of   119, 122
Ceka attachment   141, 185
CI post drills   86
Cleaning   240, 247
C. M. bar   141
Cost see Fees
Customized bars   142
Custom tray   99, 101

D

Dalla Bona   136, 139, 141, 142, 213
    advantages   213
    disadvantages   213
    laboratory procedure   213, 219
Dental examination   25
Dentition see Teeth
Diagnosis   26
Dolder bar   172, 185
    impression   172
    joint   175, 184
    laboratory procedure   172, 183
    relining   183, 185
    retention   172, 175
       adjustment of   183
Dowels
    types   89
       Schenker stepped dowel   92
       Stutz pivot   89, 92

E

Electrosurgery   66
Endodontic   36
    abutment requirements   31
    abutments   39
    access   51
    instrumentation   39, 53, 57
    medication   56
    obturation   56, 58
    therapy   36, 51, 56
    treatment plan   52, 53
    root measurement   53
    working dimensions   53, 59
EM attachment selector   136
Esthetic consideration in overdentures   21
Examination
    clinical   25
    for overdentures   25
    radiographic   26, 239
    utilization of study casts in   25, 27, 239
    visual   28

F

Fees   22, 23
Flange   71, 72
Fluoride
    gel   244
       mouthwash   244
       stannous   244

Forces see Occlusal Force
Framework design 123, 132
   coping consideration 128
     non-resilient 128
   criteria for 123
   mandibular 126
   maxillary 123
     major connector 123, 125
     minor connector 126
   occlusal record 132
   retention 125
   tissue support 125

G

Gerber attachment 197, 212
   components 198
   impression technique 200, 205
   intra-occlusal records 202
   laboratory procedure 200, 207, 235, 236
     non-resilient 207
     rebasing 208
     relining 207
     resilient 202, 207
   maintenance of 207
   management of technical 199
   non-resilient 197, 199, 207
   resilient 195, 199, 205
   treatment plan 200
   waxing of 200
Gingivectomy 66, 67
Ginta attachment 136
Gmur attachment 227, 228
Grooves, retention 77, 78, 80

H

Hader bar 136, 185, 191, 193
   advantage 193
   laboratory procedure 191, 193
   rebasing 193
   relining 193
Home care procedure for preservation
of root surfaces 242, 243, 247
Hruska 229, 230
Huser attachment 142, 197
Hygiene 240
   oral 240, 241, 244

I

IC attachment 136, 139, 141, 143, 234, 238
   laboratory procedure 236, 238
Impressions
   articulation of 106
   custom tray technique 99, 101
   hydrocolloid 102
   polyether 102
   pouring of casts 102, 105
   record bases 106
     framework record bases 107
     resin bases 106
     shellac record 106
   silicone 102
   substructure positioned 102
Interim overdentures,
   need for 32
Introfix attachment 197, 227
Ipsoclip attachment 136, 139, 142, 231, 232, 236, 237
   laboratory procedure 232-234

J

Jaw Relation records 21
   centric occlusal record 21
Jaw Relations records-cont'd
   functionally generated path record 22
     anterior guidance 108
     centric occlusion 108
     study casts 108
   incisal guidance 21
   plane of occlusion 21
   programmed cuspal inclinations

L

Long copings 46, 47
   telescopic overdenture 45
     stability 45
     retention 45
   resin denture base 46
   metal overlay coping 47
   relation to alveolar support 50

M

Maintenance of overdentures
   problems encountered 23

Major connector 126
Medium copings 48
M. F. channels 141
Mini-Zest attachment 153
Minor connector 126
Metal base
   coping relief 128
   esthetic consideration in design 129
   flange 126
   functional generated path 132
   maxillary design determination 123, 124
   mandibular design determination 127, 130
   overdenture
      non-resilient 128
      resilient 128
   retention 129, 132
   saddle area 128
Modification of existing prosthesis 69, 74
Multiple copings 113

N

Nutritional guidance 244
Non-vital abutments
   interim overdentures 72
   medium-short preparation 77

O

Overdentures
   abutment evaluation 26
      selection of 26
   abutments, criteria for 26
      available teeth 29
      bone support 27
      location of 26, 27
      masticatory load 29
      opposing dentition 29
      proximal space 20
   advantages of 20
   alveolar bone preservation 17
   attachment fixation
      advantages of 135
      disadvantages 135
   basic designs
      bare roots 133
      indications for 133
      disadvantages 133
   cleaning 240
   clinical procedure 146, 152
   construction fabrication 72, 73

coping design 148, 149
definition of 9
denture teeth 151
diagnosis 26
disadvantages 22
esthetic commitment 21
examination 25
   clinical 25
   patient history 25
   radiographic 26
   study casts 25
fee consideration 22
flasking of 73
framework design 123
home care 43
impressions for 149, 150
   master cast 150, 151
interim overdenture 69
   function of 69
Overdentures-Cont'd
   immediate 73
   maintenance
      problems encountered 23, 239, 241
   mandibular design 126
   master impressions 42
   modification of existing
      prosthesis 69, 71, 76
      with non-vital abutment 72
      with vital abutment 72
   maxillary 123
      all-metal palate 125
      horseshoe 124
   occlusal forces 29
   occlusal records 149, 150
   occlusal registration 142
   occlusion stability 21
   overlay prosthesis 20, 29
      open palate 123, 124
      metal(all) palate 123-126
      proprioceptive response 22
   path of insertion 239
   periodontal consideration 126, 128
   philosophy of 10, 117
   prosthesis
      non-resilient 128, 132
      resilient 128
   rebasing 152
   relining 152
   removal of 240
   selection of teeth 26
   speech 240
   stud attachment utilization 132
   telescopic overdenture
      advantages 133, 135, 145, 146

disadvantages 135, 145
Occlusal forces
in overdentures 29
Occlusion
occlusal records 21
Octalink attachment 81, 141
Oral hygiene see Hygiene
Orientation
casts 106

P

Paralleling devices 86
Para-Post 86
drills 86, 88
parallel post canal procedure 89
pins, types of 87
posts 86
splinted 94
Para-Max pallator 86
Palates
open 22
proprioception 22
Pins
parallel technique 93
post-pin combination 94, 97
Periodontal
abutment evaluation following
surgery 41, 42
criteria for overdentures 61, 62
probe 61
surgical evaluation 65, 66
surgical requirement 31
Periodontics
treatment plan 39, 41
abutment preparation 41
abutment selection criteria 41
electrosurgery 66
endodontics 41
fabrication of interim overdenture 41
initial operative procedure 62, 63
post surgery impression 42
diagnostic consideration 61
transitional overdentures 67
Plunger attachments
IC attachment 136, 139, 141, 143
Ipsoclip 136, 139, 142, 143
Presso-matic 143
Tach-E-Z 143
Presso-matic attachment 145
Primary see Copings
Proprioception response 22

R

Radiographic
examination 26
Rebasing
Dolder bar overdenture 183, 185
Hader bar overdenture 193
telescopic overdenture 152, 153
Zest overdenture 169, 171
Gerber overdenture 207
Record bases
functional generated occlusal
technique 107, 111
Relining
Dolder bar overdenture 183, 185
Gerber stud overdenture 207
Hader bar overdenture 183, 185
Rotherman overdenture 223, 227
telescopic overdenture 152
Zest overdenture 169, 171
Relining jig 212
Replacement
Zest male post 171
Resin record base 106
Retention 183
overdentures 183
Dalla Bona 213
Dolder bar 183
Gerber 199
Rotherman 227
Root
canals see Endodontic therapy
fluoride and surface solubility 244
reduction 36
Rotherman attachment 136, 219, 227
advantage 220
disadvantage 223
laboratory procedure 219, 221
non-resilient 219, 221
relining 223
resilient 219, 221, 224
rebasing 223
soldering 222

S

Schenker stepped dowel 92
Schubiger attachment 229, 232, 235
indication for 229
laboratory procedure 231
modification gerber 231
Screws 136, 139, 143, 144, 229
Schubiger 143, 144, 229, 230

VK-screw   144
Shellac record base   106
Sensation see Proprioceptive response 22
Silicone see Impression   102
Stud   136, 138
  indication for   138
  selection criteria   142, 195
    Ancrofix   197, 226
    Bona-puffer   228
    Ceka   197
    Dalla Bona   197
    Gerber   197
    Gmur   197
    Huser   197
    Intrafix   197
    non resilient   197
    resilient   195
    Rotherman   197
    Schubiger   197
Stutz Pivot attachment   89, 92
Surgery
  criteria for   63, 64
  treatment plan   62

T

Treatment
  planning   31-41
    endodontic rationale   32
    periodontal evaluation 32, 33, 239
    sequence plan   33-34
Tach-E-Z attachment   143
Teeth
  management of sensitivity   68

V

Vacuum process
  copings   121
VK-screw   144

W

Waxing
  coping patterns   119, 121

X

X-Ray see Radiographic

Z

Zest anchor   136, 137, 153, 172
  components   153, 154
  direct   163, 167
    gold coping procedure 165, 167
  function   153
  indirect fabrication   155, 163
  Mini-zest   167, 169
  rebasing   169, 171
  relining   169, 171
  replacement   171

Practice and Science in Dentistry

quintessence books

Shillingburg / Hobo / Whitsett

Fundamentals of Fixed Prosthodontics (Second Edition)

While retaining emphasis on basic principles, the thoroughly revised second edition features added chapters dealing with Fluid Control and Soft Tissue Management and The Functionally Generated Path Technique. Much new has been added in the discussions of techniques and materials related to porcelain, copings, and wax patterns. Nearly 200 additional illustrations supplement more than 550 from the first edition; 138 additional references are provided, some of them less than 6 months old.

   Most chapters have been expanded to make this widely acclaimed book still more useful for the practicing dentist.

454 pages, 778 illustrations, size 17.5 × 24.5 cm, linen bound with gold stamping and protective cover.

ISBN 0-931386-50-0   Order FFP $38.50

Johnson / Stratton

Fundamentals of Removable Prosthodontics

To achieve the greatest benefit from prosthodontic treatment, the principles of prevention must become an integral part of diagnosis. The philosophy of partial denture treatment described here includes patient motivation toward maintenance of oral hygiene, mouth preparation, appropriate distribution of functional stress, selection of the cleanest designs, exclusion of unnecessary elements, and striving to avoid complete edentulousness for the patient.

504 pages, 458 illustrations, size 17.5 × 24.5 cm, linen bound with gold stamping and protective cover.

ISBN 0-931386-10-1   Order JS $46.00

Practice and Science in Dentistry

quinte//ence books

Dolder/Durrer

The Bar Joint Denture

When your patient faces a "5-minutes-to-midnight" condition, when he's at risk of losing his last remaining teeth, that's the time to consider the possibility of the bar joint denture. This book, written by the developer of the Dolder bar and one of the most enthusiastic users of the technique, is based on clinical, practical experience with hundreds of patients. Clearly illustrated, the book is a manual for the use of the bar joint denture, and includes clear, unequivocal descriptions of chairside and dental laboratory techniques.

The bar-joint denture is neither experimental nor controversial; when its use is appropriate—and that's quite frequently—the bar joint denture preserves the patient's remaining teeth, and affords retention and stability simply unattainable with other techniques.

---

112 pages, 154 illustrations with 81 in color, size 17.5 × 24.5 cm, linen bound with gold stamping and protective cover.

ISBN 0-931386-02-0

Order DG $42.00

DuBrul/Menekratis

The Physiology of Oral Reconstruction

The performance of oral reconstruction aims to rectify a defective oral apparatus such as to produce a properly functional oral system. This book should be amply rewarding to anyone practicing oral care since it illuminates the inseparable interrelation between biologic function and acceptable clinical manipulation.

Structure and function are also inseparable. They simply represent the two sides of a working entity. But the behavior of a *whole* system cannot be predicted from the function of its several parts. The failure to appreciate the functional integration of the parts has led to clinical conclusions which, though they may seem obvious in superficial view are, in fact, fundamentally false.

This text is a single treatise designed in two parts. Thus it first explains the biomechanics of the oral apparatus based on the most relevant research, and then presents concepts of clinical management stemming from these critical advances. The style steers clear of wordy ramblings on unsupported notions; it is as crisp and brief as possible to reduce any haziness in communication.

---

144 pages, many illustrations with some in color, size 17.5 × 24.5 cm, linen bound with gold stamping and protective cover.

ISBN 0-931386-47-0

Order DM $42.00
